D0877857

OLD ENOUGH TO FEEL BETTER
A MEDICAL GUIDE FOR SENIORS

OLD ENOUGH TO FEEL BETTER

A MEDICAL GUIDE FOR SENIORS

MICHAEL GORDON, M.D.,
FRCP(C), FACP

 FLEET BOOKS, TORONTO

Published in 1982 by Fleet Publishers
A Division of International Thomson Limited
1410 Birchmount Road
Scarborough, Ontario, Canada M1P 2E7

ISBN 0-7706-0032-8

Published simultaneously in the United States of America
by Chilton Book Company
Chilton Way, Radnor, PA. 19089, U.S.A.

ISBN 0-8019-6991-3 *hardcover*
ISBN 0-8019-6992-1 *paperback*

Published in hardcover in 1981

Library of Congress Catalog Card No. 80-70351

A Frank E. Taylor Book

Designed by Jean Callan King/Visuality

Drawings by Lynn Waldo

Printed and bound in the United States of America

82 83 84 85 86 87 88   7 6 5 4 3 2 1

This book is dedicated to my parents and grandparents who not only enriched my life, but continually encouraged my desire to study and to teach others what I have learned.

CONTENTS

CONTENTS

FOREWORD

The history of medicine has some fairy-tale qualities. Once upon a time there was no penicillin and two-thirds of the population died of infectious diseases. Once upon a time we couldn't identify the causative organisms of tuberculosis, pneumonia, malaria, diphtheria, polio, typhoid fever or leprosy. Uncontrolled epidemics wiped out entire communities.

What we often call the "golden age of medical discovery" began in about 1870. Pasteur discovered that bacteria cause infection and Lister introduced antiseptic surgery. They opened the door on an era that has produced more medical advances than any other in history; not only were many diseases neutralized or eradicated, but the infant mortality rate has plummeted and the life expectancy rate rises yearly. With modern medicine's compendium of sophisticated treatments and techniques, many who might have died in infancy now live into old age.

But the health care needs of one segment of the population have been neglected. While childhood diseases have been nearly eradicated, and major advances are being made in treatments for cancer and other mid-life afflictions, there is a paucity of research on the health patterns of older adults. In fact, a great many questions about geriatric health and illness remain unanswered: What is normal physiology for an older person? Are the frequent short periods of sleep exhibited by many older adults an anomaly or a natural concomitant of aging? What are the effects of pollution on older adults, who often have a lower oxygen-carrying capacity? Do changes in activities and lifestyle started in the later years actually produce benefits? But perhaps the most important question is, can we do for health in the last stage of life what we have done in earlier stages: Can we eradicate the disabilities and handicaps caused by arthritis, heart disease and vision and hearing impairments? Can we identify those mental and physical capacities that *improve* with age? Can we distinguish normal decline, due to the aging process, from that which can be ameliorated, and lay to rest the myth of senility and inevitable disability?

Dr. Michael Gordon addresses these kinds of questions and argues that the older population does not have to and, indeed, *should not,* accept the stereotypical notion that old age is inevitably linked to disability and dysfunction. *Old Enough to Feel Better* marks the frontier of a redefinition of old age. It demystifies the body and provides solid information for seniors and their families that will help them become more enlightened about health and more demanding of quality care from the medical establishment. It reinforces the trend toward more patient responsibility, and encourages peer support for new health habits.

Organizations such as the Gray Panthers and Senior Olympics, and the millions of volunteers who run NRTA-AARP programs throughout the country, are living examples of an alternate vision of old age. Dr. Gordon reinforces this vision, and shines a beacon toward the day that we will be able to say: Once upon a time almost all old people suffered from arthritis, osteoporosis, and other painful diseases; once upon a time, seniors were not considered to be a vital, integral part of American life—but see how all that has changed!

Jutta Hagner
Senior Program Specialist
National Retired Teachers' Association —
American Association of Retired Persons

PREFACE

Remember the old saying, "You're old enough to know better," as though some magic wisdom automatically came with age. Throughout our lives we think of *other* people as being older, until gradually it becomes clear that *we* have become those other people. At first it may come as a shock, but eventually, individually, we must confront the reality of our aging.

We would all like to assume that as we grow older we will be treated with dignity and respect, the rewards for a long, productive, active life. We would all like to believe that we will be attended with care and consideration by members of the health profession. Unfortunately, this is not always so.

This book will give you the knowledge and understanding of your health needs necessary to make maximum use of all medical services. Your best guarantee of good health care is a sound comprehension of how your body works and how to keep it functioning well—and what happens when it is affected by illness.

With this information, plus your own determination, you will be able to ensure that your physician and all others involved in your health care respect and respond to your individual needs. Indeed, you will find that you *are* old enough to feel better.

ACKNOWLEDGMENTS

I would like to thank the many people who helped me complete this book. My association with Baycrest Centre for Geriatric Care and Mt. Sinai Hospital in Toronto gave me the experience on which much of this work is based. Steven Rudin, the executive director of Baycrest Centre, was most encouraging during all stages of the work. He supported my efforts with kind words as well as with secretarial staff and technical facilities.

I am grateful for the enthusiastic assistance of my secretaries, Rheta Fanizza and Belle Ganzon, who diligently and tirelessly worked on the manuscript until it was in its final form. Sheila Proctor and Bess Lokach of the medical records department of Baycrest Centre also earned my appreciation for their assistance during this project.

I am deeply indebted to my father, Max Gordon, and to Dr. Peter Newman, who read and reread the text and recommended changes that were crucial to the final form. Their dauntless efforts were essential to complete this work. Professor Charles Stickney and my dear aunt, Professor Marion Levine, made important contributions during the project's inception.

A vote of thanks goes to my editor, Frank E. Taylor, who believed in me when the manuscript was in infant form and helped me nurture it to maturity.

I wish to acknowledge the stimulation that I got from the Canadian Broadcasting Company's show "From Now On" and its producer, Laura Buchanan, who gave me the challenging opportunity to bring information on health care to Canada's older population. The enthusiasm of the viewing audience confirmed my belief that writing this book was a worthwhile project.

Finally, I wish to thank all my patients and friends from Baycrest Centre, Mt. Sinai Hospital, and the city of Toronto, who are a constant source of stimulation and satisfaction in my medical practice and teaching.

OLD ENOUGH TO FEEL BETTER

INTRODUCTION

How many times have you been asked, "How old are you?" Perhaps it would make more sense to ask, "How old do you feel?" It is common to place everyone above the age of 60 or 65 in that community called "senior citizens." But why was the age of 60 or 65 chosen so arbitrarily as the age for retirement? Perhaps the initial intentions behind the decision to remove older people from active participation in the work force were good ones. Unfortunately, in many cases retirement is emotionally and physically disastrous.

Older people are capable of contributing to the community, so each one of us is affected very deeply by society's edict that we remain idle and, hence, useless.

As more and more people live into their seventies and eighties and nineties with good health, sharp minds, and productive capacities, society will perhaps eventually recognize the talents of the elderly. Andrés Segovia, at the age of 88, and Vladimir Horowitz, at the age of 76, still enthrall musical audiences. The great British philosopher Bertrand Russell was mentally active and productive until his death at the age of 98. Comedian George Burns fills movie theaters at the age of 84. Charles de Gaulle and Golda Meir were politically active and respected until their deaths. At the age of 88, the loss of Marshall Tito of Yugoslavia has international repercussions. And nobody would have thought of retiring Albert Einstein at the age of 65, which would have been eleven years before his death. Like these great people, there are hundreds of thousands of elderly people who are productive and active in their own way, and, indeed, who very much want to remain so. In fact, the prospect of twenty or thirty years of inactivity may not be as conducive to good health as some of us would like to think.

The Western world has become progressively more youth-oriented. With the introduction of a mandatory retirement age and the attitudes fostered by consumerism, the older person has been placed in a nonessential role in society. The nuclear family has disintegrated, and many younger people have little experience or contact with their older parents or grandparents. If one has not related to an older individual on a personal and intimate basis, it is easy to consider all older people as uninteresting and nonproductive. Many members of the medical and nursing profession who have their major interaction with older people in hospitals, institutions, and clinics, naturally associate aging with illness.

The relative slowing down that often accompanies aging is frustrating to many younger people. It interferes with the pressure "to get things done." You only have to watch people waiting in line at a bank or ticket office when an older person is trying to carry out a transaction. The slower pace often exasperates the clerk and the younger customers waiting their turn. Have you ever noticed the impatience shown by many bus drivers for senior citizens getting on or off a bus at a pace that is too slow for the pressure of schedules? Traffic lights give little time for older persons to cross a street safely. Experiences like this can make it difficult for the older person to feel wanted and needed by the community, and it is not surprising that, once removed from an active role in the world of commerce and work, you are expected to grow old gracefully, deteriorate physically and mentally, and then pass away quietly.

It may be difficult for older people to change the attitudes of society or to have legislation initiated that will allow them to continue to be active regardless of age. However, with determination and knowledge, you can let those responsible for your health care know that you no longer accept aging as a sufficient explanation for your medical complaints. By being an informed and enlightened consumer of health care, you can direct the medical profession to respond to your needs.

The first step is to rid yourself of some of the myths that have been generated about the process of aging. If you believe the myths yourself, you will find it difficult to convince your physicians and other health personnel to discard them. I will try to give you the information that will allow you to be a well-informed recipient of health care, because a good part of the responsibility must be yours. The great tendency for older people to assign their health to their physicians puts them in a passive role about something that is crucial for positive and productive senior years. After you learn to assume the responsibility for your own health and learn to see your physician as an adviser and consultant, you will no doubt benefit both mentally and physically.

Part I of this book gives information and advice about how to use the resources and knowledge available to all of us concerning health care. Use it as a guide to assure that you get the best from the complex interaction between yourself and the medical profession. Part II is concerned with specific health problems and illnesses that may afflict you as you get older. It is the purpose of this book to enlighten you so that you can most benefit from the resources of modern medical science.

Most people assume that the inevitable process of growing old is naturally linked to illness, and this is an assumption that is shared by many members of the medical profession. It is presumed that as the body gets older, it begins to fall apart and become plagued by illness. But there is no specific age at which health deteriorates or illness occurs. To have reached your senior years, you may have survived many illnesses, or if you were extremely fortunate, perhaps you have never been ill. That you are still here is a reflection of your strength. Your age is far less important than your ability and desire to participate in life.

Frequently you will be told, "What do you expect at your age?" But, in fact, aging is not a disease. There are, of course, many illnesses that are more common in older people, but whatever illness might affect you, there are many ways to deal with it. I will try to take some of the mystery out of medicine and tell you how you can help your physician take care of you. It is less frightening and more reassuring if you know what is going on, rather than being bewildered by symptoms that are frequently puzzling and treatments that are often confusing and alarming.

Just as changes occur in childhood and adolescence, the passage from middle age to your mature years is also associated with certain changes. But these should not be thought of as illness or disease. You can continue to function very well despite these natural alterations. Many organs of the body decrease their ability to carry out functions as efficiently as you age. This gradual process begins during the early adult years and continues throughout life. Although the capacity for the body to function may decrease with age, there is ample reserve for life to continue actively and productively for many years.

As more research is done on the process of aging, it is becoming clear that some of the decline is as much a consequence of poor body maintenance as the aging process itself. A Rolls Royce will deteriorate if not properly serviced, and a Model T Ford can be kept running beautifully and efficiently if maintained with care. Although illness occurs at all ages, often without apparent reason, many of the diseases affecting older people are at least partially if not completely the result of poor health-care habits throughout a lifetime. Some of these processes can be halted or modified, if not reversed. It is in your power to make the best out of what you have. It is never too late to change, and a conversion to a more positive, active role in your own care can lead not only to better health, but to more enjoyment and satisfaction from life.

There are two sides to every medical interaction: The giver and the receiver. After you have learned more about your body and the changes or illnesses that can occur, you should be able to approach your physician intelligently and assertively. You will learn that you should receive an explanation about your medical condition. And you will find out that, whatever the illness, the possibilities of diagnosis and treatment should not be automatically denied because of your years.

It is important for you to feel comfortable with your physician. The best relationships are those that have been built up over many years. However, this is not always possible, and, unfortunately, many older people are intimidated by physicians. If you are not happy with the way your physician relates to you, do not be afraid to tell him. Some people go from one physician to another because they are afraid to tell each one that they are unhappy with their health care. This practice often leads to the absolutely worst medical care, because it takes mutual trust between physician and patient for the health care process to succeed.

Your physician should respond to your knowledge and interest positively. You should tell him that you would like to play an active role in your own health care. You can assist by confirming your confidence in his abilities. At the same time, you must express your desire to be treated honestly and openly. If you can reach this agreement with your physician, you are already well on the road to receiving good medical care.

PART ONE

A Guide to Health and Aging

CHAPTER 1

You and Your Physician

YOUR NEXT DOCTOR'S APPOINTMENT

Many people assume that because of a physician's expertise, he will be able to solve their problems quickly just by looking at them. Part of a physician's skill, however, involves extracting information and analyzing it against previous experience. Therefore, when you see your physician, you should be prepared to supply him with as much data as possible so that he can effectively analyze both your previous and present health problems.

All too often we go to a physician in mental and physical disarray, and this is often even more true as we age. Dozens of questions that you wanted to ask your physician during the preceding weeks or months suddenly elude you at the time of the interview, when emphasis may be directed to more immediate problems. Some questions may go unanswered, and you will leave feeling dissatisfied and often angry at yourself or at the physician because you did not receive a complete checkup.

Although there is no such thing as a "complete" checkup, certain parts of your medical history and physical examination will assure the likelihood of an accurate assessment of your problems. But all the poking and probing in the world cannot take the place of a well-structured interview with your physician. You can help yourself by knowing your own medical history and directing the physician to your concerns.

The center of good medical care *is* your family physician. Whether you choose a general practitioner or an internist committed to *primary care* (continuous or ongoing care), it is important to establish a good relationship. Some older people who have always enjoyed good health think that it is not necessary to have a physician until they feel ill. However, your physician should get to know you while you are well so that he has a chance to understand your personality and emotional needs before an illness occurs. This also gives him an opportunity to discuss preventive health measures with you and give advice at a time when you are not preoccupied with illness.

If you have not been to a doctor in years or if you have moved, you may have to ask friends and relatives to recommend one, or you can call your city or county medical society. Many medical centers have departments of family and community medicine that can also help. When you go to a new physician, explain to him *how* you would like to be involved in your own health care and be sure that you understand each other.

One usually sees a physician either for a routine checkup, to follow up on an illness or treatment, or because something unexpected has happened. In any of these situations it is important that you document the events that have occurred since your last appointment. You should also make a note to tell the physician of any other medical people you have seen, as well as any medications you have received.

If something *new* has happened since your last visit, you should record the sequence of events from the beginning of the *new* symptom. For example, you may have had a dizzy spell and thought nothing of it. A week later you had another spell and almost fell. You make an appointment with your physician for two weeks hence, and during this time you have two further spells, one of which actually causes a fall where you bump your head.

To complicate matters, you are taking two medications to control your blood pressure, but you decide to change the medication yourself because you think your blood pressure is too high or too low. Perhaps you have received this advice from a relative or neighbor or from a nurse or doctor at the emergency room, where you went for treatment of your head injury. By the time you see your physician, a month may have passed since your first dizzy spell. The sequence of events may now be vague or even forgotten, and the changes in medication also may have become mixed up. Trying to recall this sequence of events accurately when questioned by your physician can be frustrating to both of you.

The point is that you should always spend a few minutes prior to the appointment to write down the date, time, and circumstances of each event. Each one should be described and the exact changes in medication or dosage recorded. If, for example, the doctor at the emergency room said your blood pressure was 150/80, write it down, as well as the name of the doctor and the emergency room. Also, bring all prescription drugs that you were given so that the physician can check the type of medication and dosage to make sure that there has been no mix-up.

When the visit is for a follow-up examination and nothing new has happened since the previous appointment, it is usually easier to remember what events have occurred in the mean-time. However, variations in the effects of previously prescribed treatments should be noted in writing and *all medications in their original containers should be brought to the physician for examination. A list* of pills or unbottled samples is not enough. Innumerable errors can occur even when you think you know your pills. This is especially the case with the many drug benefit programs for the elderly that often require that equivalent (generic) medications be given instead of trade names.

For example, an alert, intelligent 80-year-old patient came to me for a follow-up visit. She suffered from heart failure and knew that she took *digoxin* for her heart, *furosemide* for her "water," and *diazepam* for sleep. There were no new complaints about her exercise tolerance, breathing, or chest pain. She mentioned, however, that she had difficulty sleeping because she had to go to the bathroom frequently at night. She also had difficulty getting around in the morning because she was very drowsy. The three bottles of pills were clearly labeled as to the contents and dosage; all three were small yellow pills. She had initially written on the bottle caps: *Morning* on the digoxin, *Morning* on the furosemide, and *Bedtime* on the diazepam.

It so happened that the bottle caps were identical, and inadvertently they had been switched. Therefore, she was taking furosemide before bedtime and diazepam in the morning. Fortunately, her heart failure did not suffer from this mix-up, and her symptoms were easily cured by putting the right bottle caps on the right bottles. If she had brought only a list or sample of the pills instead of the pills in their original containers, the problem would not have been so easily solved.

Another example is that of an elderly man who was brought to me by his daughters because they felt he was becoming senile. He was confused at times and occasionally staggered when he walked. They thought perhaps that he needed to be put in a nursing home. My examination revealed nothing to suggest memory loss. However, he complained bitterly that his laxative was no longer working. He said that sometimes he took one or two capsules a day and would not have a bowel movement.

He produced his medications, including the "laxative." This proved to be a sleeping capsule, which was the same color as the laxative. The laxative had been discarded by mistake instead of his sleeping medications, which he had discontinued three weeks earlier. The patient had been taking one or two of these sleeping capsules daily in order to move his bowels, which, of course, did not happen. They did, however, cause him to become confused and have difficulty walking. This was cured by disposing of the sleeping pills and giving him a new prescription for the laxative.

You are not the only one who might make an error in the dosage of medications. Although special precautions are taken, pharmacies can make mistakes. A 70-year-old lady showed me her bottle of digoxin, which she was taking for her heart. She complained of loss of appetite. According to my records, she was supposed to be taking one small yellow pill. The bottle contained a small white pill, which was the same medication but in twice the strength. The label on the bottle said that the contents were the smaller size. An error had been made at the pharmacy. When the dosage was adjusted to the smaller amount, her appetite returned to normal.

Many equivalent drugs are called by different names and even *look* different. In fact, you may receive one prescription from one physician and another from a second physician or from a hospital or clinic. The best way to assure that the drugs are not getting mixed up is to bring all of them in their original containers whenever you visit your physician. This is even more important if many changes have been made in the medication since it was originally prescribed. It is amazing how many drugs can be discontinued or decreased after your physician has a chance to check all of them.

HOW TO PRESENT YOUR SYMPTOMS

Many older people have great difficulty explaining their symptoms to their physician. Sometimes it is a problem in communication, and sometimes the difficulty lies in the symptoms themselves, which are often less pronounced as you age. Some older people feel that the more complaints they have, the more the physician will be impressed with the seriousness of their problem. Others are stoics and do not want to "bother" him, thinking that somehow he will figure things out.

Before you visit your physician, carefully write down all of your symptoms and the order in which they occurred. Try to describe them carefully, using as many different words as possible. Some feelings are so vague that it may be difficult to put them in words. For example, feeling "weak" means different things to different people. To some it means that their muscles have less strength to carry out certain everyday activities, such as not being able to lift a bag of groceries or get up from a chair. Some use the word *weakness* when they really mean shortness of breath, while others mean that they have no motivation to do routine chores. If you elaborate just what it is that you cannot do because of this "weakness," your physician will be able to determine the reason more quickly.

Many symptoms and complaints are common in the older person. Because you may have only one of them does not mean that it is natural and can be disregarded. In general, any new, unusual symptom should be reported to your physician. In many cases complaints may be the result of something minor and temporary, but be sure to tell him so that proper steps are taken to deal with them.

Some complaints may arise from an unknown illness, and it may take time for all the pieces to fit together and a diagnosis made. For example, you find that you occasionally have shortness of breath. One day, along with the shortness of breath, you suddenly become dizzy and almost fall. You make an appointment to see your physician. During the next few days you have some chest pain that precedes the dizziness and shortness of breath. The attacks begin to come so often that you feel too weak to carry out your normal activities. By the time you see your physician or go to a hospital emergency room, you have had a few sleepness nights because of difficulty in breathing.

In another instance you might notice that your appetite is poor. Your family comments that you are picking at your food, and you find that your clothes are looser because you have lost weight. When you wake up in the morning, you see that your pajamas are wet, and when you measure your temperature at night, you discover that you have a fever. Before you are able to see your doctor, you have developed diarrhea or abdominal pain.

In these instances the exact illness may not be clear from the first complaint. Shortness of breath, dizziness, and chest pain can be the first signs of heart disease. *Weakness* is a vague term, but in the context of the other complaints, it takes on a special meaning. Poor appetite and weight loss can have many causes. However, when diarrhea and abdominal pain are present, certain kinds of illnesses should be considered.

Remember, you are the key that allows the physician to interpret your symptoms. So always be prepared to describe them as accurately as possible.

THE PHYSICAL EXAMINATION

We assume that when we see a physician, we will be given a physical examination. However, it is usually not necessary for you to be examined fully at every appointment. Many physicians will do a complete physical examination semiannually or annually. At other times, a routine examination may include listening to your heart and lungs, measuring blood pressure and perhaps examining a part of your body that has caused recent concern.

If a physician never examines you completely, you should ask why. If an appointment for a complete examination is not then arranged, you might consider changing physicians. A full examination requires that you undress completely, so wear garments to the doctor's office that can be easily removed without assistance. Wear a simple dress or trousers with zippers, and tops with short sleeves or very wide sleeves so that the chest and arms can be easily examined. Corsets and girdles should be avoided. Often the abdomen is overlooked because it is encased in a girdle that takes ten minutes to remove. Stockings that can be easily taken off, or none at all, make it easier for the physician to examine your feet. This is important because as you get older, your feet need to be examined more often.

The physician usually starts with one part of the body and works his way along, examining the different organs and systems. Many older people are upset by an examination of the rectum. This is first done with a finger, then with an instrument called a *proctoscope* or *sigmoidoscope,* which allows the physician to see the lower end of the bowel. Many older women are embarrassed by a vaginal examination and often feel that at their age it is no longer necessary. However, you should allow the physician to examine the whole body, including the rectum and vagina, even though it may be uncomfortable. In fact, if your physician has *never* examined these parts, ask him to do so.

If you have not had a complete examination for more than a year, make an appointment to have one. Be prepared to undress completely. It is well worth the time and effort.

YOUR FAMILY AND YOUR PHYSICIAN

As you grow older, you may become more dependent on members of your family. Whereas you may have gone to a doctor's appointment on your own for years, you may begin to feel more secure if you go with your spouse or with one of your children. Sometimes a member of your family first convinces you to see your physician for symptoms that you may not be aware of or consider important.

When you go to your physician with a member of your family, decide beforehand just what you expect from him and from your family member. Children and spouses sometimes tend to "take over," thereby preventing you from making your own decisions. It is common for children to assume the role of parent to their own parents as time goes on. This is even more true when one of the parents has died and the remaining one becomes more dependent on children.

You should discuss openly and honestly what role you would like your family to take in your health care. If you feel competent, insist that all decisions be made only with your approval and understanding. In addition, clarify this point with your physician or any other physicians who become involved in your care. Family members and physicians often assume that older people are not capable of or interested in making decisions about their own health. This can lead to serious difficulties and errors in judgment that can affect you directly.

Although I have had similar experiences with much younger people, I recall vividly the case of an energetic 90-year-old woman who was referred to me because of abdominal discomfort and weight loss. I had seen her on a number of previous occasions for other medical problems. At this time she was sent to me because an abdominal X-ray showed a suspicious area in her stomach.

We had previously agreed that I would be honest and direct with her. The X-ray suggested an ulcer, but the report questioned whether it might be malignant. She had not responded to some simple ulcer treatment, and the referring physician asked for my opinion. I explained to the patient that she probably had an ulcer, but because it was not healing as quickly as normally expected, we should investigate it further with a *gastroscopy*. After I explained the procedure and answered her questions, she agreed to the test.

Later that day, I received an urgent phone call from her angry son, who was upset and annoyed that I had discussed her condition and the test with her before I had conferred with him. I told him that his mother was perfectly capable of understanding her medical condition and making her own decisions. He was furious because he felt that "at her age" she could not possibly know what was going on.

The day before the test, I again spoke to the patient. She once more confirmed her desire to make her own decisions. I asked her to tell her family how she felt because they obviously were not aware of her wishes or her capabilities. The test proved that the ulcer was benign, and more intensive therapy resulted in a cure.

There is nothing wrong with having a family member accompany you to your doctor's appointment. Often, a family member can supply additional information about your symptoms. For instance, if you have had a number of fainting spells, a witness may be able to provide information that will help diagnose the cause. If the instructions given by the doctor are complex, another family member can reinforce the instructions to you. Having the physician write down complicated instructions is also valuable.

Try to remain independent with the doctor, however. For instance, you can request a private and personal medical interview without your children or spouse being in the same room. This allows you to express any personal problems and conflicts that you may be experiencing with your family. If you wish to have your children or spouse present during the interview, tell your physician. Some time alone with your doctor, however, is very important. On the other hand, it may also be useful for your family to have some time with the doctor to confirm problems or add information, but this should never be requested unless you have had the same opportunity.

Your physician should gauge your ability to answer your *own* questions. Family members often tend to compensate and "fill in" deficiencies in a failing memory. Too much interference by your family can make the interview less productive. Remember that they are there to help you, but it is still *your* appointment. It is understandable to want to confer with family members before agreeing to tests or treatments. However, make it clear that the final decision is to be yours after you have received their advice.

The time may come when you may be incapable of making your own decisions. You may be unconscious because of a disease or an accident or have an illness that interferes with your decision-making ability. Make a point of discussing with close family members your desires about your health and life while you are well, rather than having them assume the decisions for you. Learn to be direct with your family and open with your physician so that your own best interests will always be protected whenever decisions concerning you have to be made.

When your family has to make choices on your behalf, it is better if you have built up a feeling of trust over the years. This way they will feel comfortable doing their best for you. The help of a social worker experienced in the care of the elderly can be useful in assisting in decisions concerning institutionalization or other such problems. A sympathetic physician, preferably one who has known you and your family for some time, also can be helpful.

PRESCRIPTION AND OVER-THE-COUNTER DRUGS

Your physician will often prescribe at least the occasional use of medications. How you use medications, both prescription and nonprescription, can have a major effect on your health.

As many of us commonly do, older people tend to keep drugs that they are no longer using, and they may take them at a later time without instructions from a physician. You may share the common tendency for self-diagnosis and self-treatment and may try medications that have been given to you by relatives or neighbors. And with Medicare and similar social and drug benefit programs, duplicate drugs may be dispensed under different names. You might not be aware that you are taking more than the prescribed amount because it has come in two different bottles with two different names.

Recently, I saw an older woman who complained of weakness, fatigue, and memory loss. She was taking Valium® and two *generic* (chemical or official name) drugs that were exactly the same but dispensed by different pharmacies. Therefore, she was taking three times the prescribed dosage. When the drugs were stopped, she perked up and her symptoms disappeared.

19

Always ask that the *generic* name be printed on the label even if the *trade* name appears.

When a physician prescribes a medication, he has weighed its likely benefits and the possible risks. When you receive a prescription, you and your family should make sure that you understand for how long the medication is to be taken and under what circumstances it might be stopped.

In many instances a supply of medication is given for a month at a time. You may not be aware that when the prescription is finished, it has to be renewed. This should be clarified before the prescription is filled and the instructions carefully discussed with your physician and pharmacist.

As you grow older, your body's ability to dispose of excess medication decreases. The liver and kidneys weaken, which means the drugs are eliminated from the body more slowly. Therefore, the dosage that you require of a drug is frequently smaller than that for a younger person, and the period between doses may be longer. Your physician takes this into account when he prescribes a drug for you.

Many people take more than one medication simultaneously. Different drugs can interfere with each other, or certain combinations of drugs cause one drug to become inactive. An interaction can also lead to an increase in the side effects from one of the medications. Whenever a drug is prescribed, inform your physician of all other medications that you are taking. Make sure that there are no special precautions that must be observed with the new drug when it is added to the others.

When you take more than one medication, you may assume that the different kinds of pills cannot be swallowed at the same time. But in most instances, many medications *can* be taken together. Your body deals with each one separately once it enters your stomach. Otherwise it could be a nightmare to take four kinds of tablets four times each day and take them all separately!

However, certain medications *cannot* be taken together. For example, antacids interfere with the absorption of iron pills.

Some medications should be taken on an empty stomach; others are best tolerated when taken after meals. If many medications are involved, discuss with your physician when they should be taken. This will assure that the best effects of the drugs are achieved.

To ensure that you are taking your medications correctly, take all your medications in their original bottles when you visit a physician or go to a hospital. Your physician can then check if the prescriptions have been filled properly and if there has been any inadvertent duplication. Or when you are discharged from the hospital, new prescriptions may be written that may duplicate the drugs already being taken. The new directions should be gone over carefully with the doctor before you go home.

Everyone has become very conscious and afraid of drug side effects. When you receive a prescription from your physician, discuss any side effects before you leave the office. Although many medications have side effects, the probable benefit of the drug is usually much greater than the side effects. Should a serious side effect occur, discontinue the medication and inform your physician immediately. He may substitute another medication or instruct you how to decrease or treat the side effect. In general, it is safer to stop a medication causing a side effect rather than treat it with another medication, unless the initial drug is crucial to your health and there is no substitute. However, never stop the medication without discussing it with your physician first. You could miss important therapy.

Many people of all ages buy *over-the-counter* (or patent) drugs, meaning that they require no prescription. This usually implies self-diagnosis and self-treatment, which has a greater potential for danger as you grow older. For the occasional symptom that is relieved easily, self-treatment is acceptable. However, prescription medications and those bought over the counter may interact adversely.

Except for an occasional pain reliever or antacid, over-the-counter medications are not recommended. Some cold mixtures, for example, contain antihistamines, which when taken with other medications can cause serious side effects. Decongestant tablets and eye drops bought without prescription can affect your blood pressure.

An elderly woman was recently admitted to the hospital in a coma. Her family said her speech had become slurred the day before hospitalization. She also complained that she was going deaf. The family thought she had had a stroke, when, in fact, she was ultimately found to be suffering from aspirin poisoning. When she woke up, she said she had been taking eight or ten Anacin® tablets a day for her back pain during the previous week. Anacin®, like Bufferin®, Alka Seltzer®, and many other medications, contain aspirin. She did not realize that the eight "brown pills" that her doctor had given her to take each day for arthritis were also a kind of aspirin. No wonder she went into coma. When she bought the Anacin®, she did not ask anyone, including her pharmacist, if they could be taken with her prescription pills.

Whenever possible, you should receive your medications by prescription, and always try to use the same pharmacy to fill the prescriptions. The pharmacist should keep a record of your medications and can check to see if there are any problems with the drugs and the dosages. Pharmacists can warn you about the inappropriate use of over-the-counter medicines when they know your prescription drugs, and they can inform physicians of possible oversights or errors in prescribing.

CHAPTER 2

Specialists

Every now and then your family physician may refer you to a specialist for consultation. Or perhaps you have gone to a specialist without asking your physician, assuming that he will be upset because you want a second opinion. However, by seeing other physicians on your own, you may be doing yourself more harm than good. It is always in your best interest to have your physician coordinate your health care.

When your family physician refers you to a specialist, he will send on your behalf a summary of your problems and the results of any tests and medications. This informs the specialist of your medical history so that he knows your background in advance. Then, with the combination of information from your physician and your own personal account, he can more easily assess your difficulties. Make sure that your physician is sending the information, or ask if you should present some of the data yourself.

Whenever possible, know the reason for the referral, and ask what will be involved in the consultation. It is very distressing to find that the specialist intends to perform tests or procedures for which you have not been mentally and physically prepared. And the specialist, too, is usually equally upset when this happens. Following the visit, ask about the findings and if any tests are recommended. Some specialists will send a report to your physician, who, in turn, will inform you. Understand before leaving the specialist's office how you will receive the results of the examination.

As medicine has become more complex, numerous medical specialties have developed. Physicians are usually divided into those who practice *surgery* and those who practice *medicine.* At the center of medical care should be your own physician, who may be a family practitioner or a general practitioner. The specialist most often seen by older people is an *internist.* Unlike the general practitioner, or GP, the internist will not take on the care of children or pregnant women or do various types of minor surgery. In many parts of the world internists also act as *primary-care* physicians; in others they act as consultants to family physicians for more complex problems.

In the United States and Canada especially, but in most Western countries as well, specialists have been trained extensively in one area of medical expertise beyond their medical school training. The names used to describe the different kinds of specialists come from either Greek or Latin words that refer to the particular part of the body. The terms usually end in the suffix *ologist,* which means *one who has studied.* Therefore, a specialist of the heart is a *cardiologist, cardio* meaning *heart.* A *rheumatologist* deals with diseases of the muscles and joints, so special arthritic problems are often referred to him. *Nephrologists* treat kidney disorders, although often they take a special interest in high blood pressure as well.

A *respirologist* or *pulmonologist* is a chest specialist, mainly concerned with illnesses that affect the respiratory system. Physicians specializing in the digestive system are *gastroenterologists.* If you develop an unusual blood disorder, you may be sent to a *hematologist. Oncologists* are specially trained in treating cancer (neoplastic diseases), but they often work closely with hematologists, and frequently the two specialties are combined.

Allergists and *immunologists* are concerned with problems that lead to sensitivity (allergy) to various substances, both from within and outside the body. These specialties often overlap. A *neurologist* primarily deals with illnesses of the brain and nervous system. If you suffer from a hormonal disease, which often originates in the endocrine glands, you may be referred to an *endocrinologist.*

There are also many different surgical specialties. Depending on your particular problem, your family physician may send you to a *general surgeon* or one dealing with a special part of the body, such as a *vascular surgeon* should you have a disease of the blood vessels, or an *orthopedic surgeon* for bones requiring surgical repair. Many women are sent to *gynecologists* for disorders affecting their reproductive or urinary systems. Men may be referred to a *urologist* for similar disorders.

Many other physicians are not strictly "medical," but they are often necessary for the older person. These include *psychiatrists,* who deal with emotional problems, and *physiatrists* (physicians specializing in rehabilitation), who are concerned with rehabilitation after illness, injury, or surgery.

GERIATRICIANS

One of the newest specialties in the United States and Canada, which has long existed in other parts of the Western world, is *geriatrics.* Even though your physician may choose to send you to a number of specialists if you have multiple problems, sometimes the end result is too many cooks for the broth. This becomes more evident as people grow older and develop problems that fall into various specialties.

There is a great deal of confusion about the terms *gerontologist* and *geriatrician.* Gerontology is the study of aging, including the social, financial, biological, political, and medical influences on the aging process. A gerontologist, however, usually is not involved directly in the care of the older individual. A *geriatrician* is a physician who specializes in diagnosing and treating the elderly. The main thrust of formal geriatric training has occurred more in Europe and Great Britain than in the United States and Canada, where only recently medical schools and hospitals have developed departments of geriatric medicine.

A competent geriatric specialist usually has a degree or diploma in internal medicine and has undertaken specific further training in many aspects of the aging process. This usually includes special studies in neurology, physical therapy and rehabilitation, and psychiatry.

Because many medical problems can affect you simultaneously as you grow older, sometimes it is necessary to combine information and expertise from many medical specialties in order to reach a decision about the best health care for you. If your family physician feels that your problems are excessively complex or that you are not functioning at your best level, he may refer you to a geriatric specialist for an overall, in-depth evaluation of all your problems. He can recommend any tests and therapies that might be necessary to achieve your best level of health.

In almost every city, there are family physicians and internists who are especially interested in the care of the elderly but who do not necessarily refer to themselves as geriatricians. With the rapid increase in the number of elderly individuals in society, it has become clear that physicians specifically trained to care for older people will be needed in greater numbers. Many medical schools and hospitals in the United States and Canada are investing money and effort in geriatric training programs and the development of geriatric departments.

Within the next few years it should become increasingly possible for a family physician to find a geriatrician who is qualified to provide the consultative services necessary for your best care. Do not expect to be transferred to the exclusive care of such a specialist, however. In general, it is in your best interest to have your ongoing care directed by your family physician. He can rely on the assistance and advice of specialists, including that of a geriatrician, to assure you of the best care available.

SELECTING A SURGEON

Many people at sometime in their lives are faced with the possibility of surgery, and it can be an extremely frightening prospect, especially as you grow older. Sometimes necessary and important surgery may not be performed because you, your family, and even your physician assume that the risks are too great at your age, whatever it might be. Very often this is *not* true. Surgery, if likely to improve your health, should not be denied to you because of age alone.

Surgery can be done on either an *elective* or *emergency* basis. Elective surgery means that you and the surgeon have agreed that surgery is necessary, but that it can be done at a time that is convenient for both of you. For example, if it has taken two or three years for your cataract to have progressed to the point that its removal can safely and effectively improve your vision, there is no urgency to do it immediately. Surgery can be "booked" according to convenience. On the other hand, if you unexpectedly develop a retinal detachment in your eye and suddenly become blind, the more time that passes before surgery, the less likely it is that it will be successful. This would be an emergency operation.

It is important to distinguish between these two situations, because, whenever possible, the general condition of your health should be evaluated before surgery. If you are not in optimal health before an elective procedure, your physician may ask the surgeon to postpone the operation until your health improves. If, for example, your diabetes is not under control, your blood pressure too high, or if you have recently begun to experience the pain of angina pectoris, it is best to postpone elective surgery until these problems have been brought under control and your physical condition is stable.

Emergency surgery is usually recommended when your condition threatens your life or seriously affects your health. Under such circumstances it might be necessary to accept certain risks in order to achieve the benefits of surgery. The degree of urgency must be discussed with the surgeon, and often a medical assessment by a physician skilled in preparing older people for surgery is warranted. In these situations the care after surgery is very important. A team approach, with cooperation between the surgeon and your family physician or internist can be very helpful.

Some medical centers are well known for their expertise in operating on the elderly, and your physician should be able to recommend a surgeon who is well qualified to perform the kind of surgery that you require. You can check his reputation by speaking to families and patients who have been treated previously by him.

You can often tell from your interview with the surgeon whether he is especially compassionate in treating older people. His patience and attitude when speaking to you and your family may be a guide. However, this does not necessarily reflect his skill as a surgeon. That can be judged only by physicians who have previously dealt with him and patients who have been treated by him and it is enormously important to rely on those recommendations. Reputations are usually made by success, so do not be afraid to ask questions about a surgeon's experience. It is very hard to undo damage caused by surgery, so by the time you agree to an operation, you should feel confident that you have found the right surgeon for you.

Danger from surgery partially depends on the experience of the surgeon in operating on your particular problem. However, surgery on the eye for cataracts and glaucoma, surgery to repair a broken hip, prostate surgery on men, and some kinds of female gynecological surgery are commonly performed on older people. Also, insertion of a pacemaker and most surgery for vascular (blood-vessel) disease is done on older people as well. Therefore, if you have chosen your surgeon carefully, you will probably tolerate the operation with little risk.

One danger of surgery is the use of an anesthetic. Many older people are frightened by anesthesia, especially if they had surgery years ago, when anesthetic techniques were less well developed. However, modern anesthesia and *anesthesiologists* and *anesthetists* (physicians and nurses trained in anesthesia) can bring you through surgery with a remarkably small risk. As important as the surgery itself is the question of medication that may be used afterward. Dosage of drugs should be adjusted according to your age and medical condition so that difficulties and side effects are avoided. Your physician, working closely with your surgeon, will decide on the appropriate dosage.

PREPARATION FOR AN OPERATION

Probably the greatest surgical risk for older people is from problems that existed prior to the need for surgery. Those people with severe heart, lung, or brain disease will have more difficulty coming through an operation successfully than those who have been relatively healthy. The elderly individual who has severe memory impairment may also have difficulty with surgery because he is less often able to cooperate in his postsurgical care. Clearly the urgency and seriousness of the operation must be carefully weighed against your general health and the likelihood of success. You can help by maintaining your health and preparing yourself for the operation. To assure optimal health, a careful examination by your physician should be arranged. Existing medical problems should be reevaluated and treated before the operation.

If you are a smoker, you should stop smoking for at least a few weeks before the operation. Increasing your degree of physical activity with long walks and calisthenics can improve your muscle tone. It is worthwhile practicing deep breathing, coughing, and foot and leg strengthening exercises to help maintain your circulation after the operation. These measures can also help prevent pneumonia. The exercises should be explained to you by your physician before surgery in order to give you time to rehearse them. Very often a physical therapist may see you in the hospital just prior to your operation to make sure you understand your exercises, and she will help you to do them after surgery.

Before you agree to an operation, your physician should carefully explain the reasons for the surgery, its goals, and the risks involved, as well as factors that may increase the hazards. Your surgeon should explain possible complications and recommend ways to avert them. You and your family should weigh the relative risks and benefits of the surgery, although this may not be possible in an emergency situation, where prompt intervention could mean the difference between life and death. For example, if you have a hernia, there is a risk that one day it may become twisted. This would require emergency surgery, which is more hazardous than elective surgery. The possibility that an elective hernia repair will not succeed, or that complications may set in, is relatively small. If you are otherwise in good health, most physicians would recommend that your hernia be repaired, rather than run the risk of an emergency operation.

It is very important that you discuss your expectations of the surgery with your family physician and the surgeon. Unless you really understand the likely results, you may be disappointed, which will upset you as well as the surgeon. If you think that a surgical operation is being done to relieve pain, but the surgeon is doing it for another reason, you will be disappointed to discover that the pain persists after the surgery. Some operations are done to *prevent* problems, so the benefit may not be apparent immediately. Therefore, it is very important that you understand the possible outcome of the operation and what kind of treatment may be required after surgery.

Older patients are often concerned about getting a second

opinion before they agree to surgery. A second opinion, how-ever, does not necessarily solve the problem as to whether or not you require surgery. What it does do is make you and your family feel more confident that the right decision is being made.

It is probably best to have the initial recommendation for surgery made by a nonsurgeon, such as your family physician or an internist. The family physician or internist who refers you should give his opinion as to whether your general state of health is sufficiently good to withstand an operation. If the surgeon agrees that surgery would be beneficial, you already have two opinions. If you have reservations, or if your physician or surgeon is doubtful, get an opinion from another physician who is not directly involved in the case. A surgeon is usually chosen by his experience with previous older patients who have required similar operations.

In certain types of specialized surgery, such as eye surgery, your family physician or internist may not be able to help you decide on surgery, other than assuring you that your *ophthalmologist* (eye doctor) is of high caliber.

Even with the best medical care and an outstanding surgeon, with every operation there is a possibility of problems. The most obvious undesirable outcome is that the operation itself does not succeed. For example, if your cataract is to be removed, it may be removed successfully, but if your *retina* (back of the eye) is severely diseased, your vision may not improve despite successful surgery on the cataract. A bowel tumor causing a blockage may not always be removable. Blood vessels may be so poor that a bypass graft cannot be put in place because the stitches cannot be held by the diseased arteries. But remember, all surgery has risks. You must understand the relative danger of surgery, the hazards of not operating, and the likelihood of success or failure. After you have that information, *you* must decide if you will accept the recommendations and advice of your physician and surgeon.

In major surgery death is always a possibility. The more urgent the surgery, the greater the likelihood that this may happen. In elective surgery, on the other hand, you and your family may not understand that there still may be a possibility of death, however remote. This, too, should be discussed with the surgeon. With modern anesthetics and good care, the vast majority of older people can undergo surgery with a very *small* risk of not surviving the operation and the postoperative period. The risk should not keep you from agreeing to surgery that may significantly improve your life or health.

Postoperatively, some older individuals develop an infection of the urinary tract. This is more common if you have had major surgery and require a *catheter* for the drainage of urine. In most cases these infections can be adequately and successfully controlled, and it is very likely that you will respond favorably to treatment.

You may become temporarily mentally confused following surgery. This may be the result of the anesthetic or the medications used to treat pain, nausea, or vomiting. It may occur because of infections, fluid accumulation, problems with your metabolism, or the sensory deprivation that results from patching the eyes after cataract surgery. There may be a need to treat infections or discontinue some medications in order to reverse the mental confusion. In almost all instances the condition is treatable, and within a few days of the operation, most patients will return to a good level of function. You will probably need a period of convalescence or rehabilitation, but if the surgery was not stressful, you could be discharged relatively soon.

Do not discount the benefits of surgery because of your age. The chances are that if you have reached an old age you are probably made of very resilient material. Use your physician as a consultant and choose the best surgeon possible.

An 85-year-old gentleman entered the hospital with a severe case of pancreatitis. He had refused to have his gall stones removed (which had caused him problems in the past) because he felt he was "too old." After much coaxing he agreed to an operation in order to prevent the risk of another attack of pancreatitis, as well as the episodes of abdominal pain from his gallbladder disease. His wife was fearful of the operation but finally agreed to it when she realized that he had almost died from his attack of pancreatitis.

His operation went smoothly. A week later when I saw him, while he was waiting to be discharged, he looked at me with a long face and said that he was very unhappy. I asked why, because I expected that he would be as delighted as I was with the successful result of his operation. He looked at me with a smile and said, "They aren't giving me enough food." Two years after his surgery, he is still vigorous and has not had an attack of abdominal pain since his operation.

COSMETIC SURGERY

We would all like to remain perpetually young. Since this is impossible, some older individuals at least try to keep their youthful appearance. Many factors contribute to feelings of youthfulness and vigor, and they are at least as important as one's cosmetic appearance.

When you are overweight, you not only appear less youthful, but also you usually cannot engage in activities that will make you feel younger. An active and vital lifestyle and good health practices are more important in making you feel and look youthful and vigorous than the removal of wrinkles from your face. However, you may feel that your outward appearance belies your true feelings of youth and interferes with your activities and interests. You may feel that if you "look" more youthful you will be able to enjoy life more fully. Under such circumstances cosmetic surgery might be suitable for you.

Many surgical operations can be done, but the most common one to enhance your features is the *surgical face-lift*. In addition, operations can be performed on the eyelids, chin, and nose.

The face-lift consists of "pulling back" the skin and underlying tissues of the face and removing the excess. The scars are usually behind the ear and under the scalp, where they will be less noticeable. During a face-lift operation, small pockets of fat that cause parts of your face to bulge may also be removed. Surgery on the eyelids usually removes excess fat and redundant skin so that your eyes do not appear to be baggy or your eyelids droopy. Some plastic surgeons may also modify the appearance of your nose as part of a facial reconstruction. Sometimes the surgeon will also either manually or chemically "peel" the skin blemishes and fine wrinkles that may make you look older.

This surgery is *not* done for the same reasons that most other surgery is performed. Your health or life is not at risk. Therefore, you should consider it carefully. And in this case a second opinion can be worthwhile. As with all surgery, complications are possible. Very few competent plastic surgeons will propose this type of surgery if your general health is poor and if you have not attempted to lose weight and improve your exercise tolerance. Even with the best surgical technique, some people may suffer from excess bleeding during surgery or have scars that do not heal well. More serious complications occur rarely, and a competent surgeon should be able to anticipate these and avoid them.

The most common problem associated with a surgical face-lift is disappointment with the outcome. Before committing yourself to this type of operation, you should discuss your expectations with the surgeon and ask him for an honest prediction of the result. Sometimes more than one surgical procedure is necessary to achieve a good result. You should discuss this with the surgeon in order to avoid the surprise and shock when he recommends another operation.

It is just as important to choose the right plastic surgeon as it is to choose any other kind of surgeon. Most major medical centers have departments of plastic surgery that are staffed by competent surgeons, and your physician and other patients can help you decide on the right one for you. In some areas there are special institutes for plastic surgery, and they usually maintain a good reputation.

After a surgical face-lift, you must do your best to keep your weight under control, because excess fat can interfere with what otherwise would have been a good outcome. Quite often, as the aging process continues, the results of the face-lift may disappear. Depending on your personality and desire to appear more youthful, you may require a second or even third face-lift a few years later.

Remember, your outward physical appearance should be only one part of your program of creative and vigorous aging. Your level of physical activity and your emotional and intellectual interests play a crucial part in making you feel youthful. Do not confuse *looking* youthful and *being* youthful. If you decide to have cosmetic surgery, make sure that you match your activities and lifestyle with your appearance.

DENTISTS AND DENTAL CARE

Unfortunately, many people do not consider their teeth to be as important to their health as other parts of their body. It is surprising just how little time many people put into dental care, although they will spend great sums of money and enormous amounts of time taking care of their "health." A recent cover of a national magazine showed a famous singer smiling and revealing teeth that were plagued by terrible gums. Without good teeth, his singing career could eventually be jeopardized.

Your dentist should be selected with as much care as your physician. You may have had the same dentist for many years and, if so, you'll want to continue with him as you grow older. Should you have to find a new dentist, it is worthwhile locating one who has a special interest in the care of the elderly. The advice of friends or the local dental society can be of value in finding a suitable dentist.

In many dental schools the curriculum is similar to medical school for the first few years; then the dentist specializes in diseases of the gums and teeth. Therefore, your dentist should be concerned with your general medical condition and aware of any health problems you may have. When you go to a dentist for the first time, he will take a medical and dental history from you. Major medical problems will influence the choice of anesthetic used, whether antibiotics will be needed, and what kind of painkillers might be required after treatment.

Your dentist and physician should communicate about your medical problems, and you should inform your dentist of your illnesses. With your physician's help, he can treat you without danger to your health.

Your teeth are very important. Even though you are no longer growing physically, proper nutrition is still important. A balanced diet ensures normal bodily functions and repair after injury, and it maintains your body's defenses against disease. Without good teeth and gums, it is difficult to achieve good nutrition. Foods cannot be chewed properly and digestion may be impaired. Your teeth are important for other reasons too. They help the tongue in the process of swallowing food, and they are essential in speaking properly. People without good teeth are often poorly understood. Your speech problem may be misinterpreted and thought to be psychological or neurological.

Your teeth are also important to your appearance. If you have lost your teeth, your facial muscles will become distorted, which will make you appear older than your age. Consequently, you may not want to be seen without dentures. If you lose your dentures, you may foolishly even consider going into seclusion until they are replaced.

Older people tend to have poor dental health for numerous reasons. For many, unfortunately, poor dental care is a lifelong habit. As a child and young adult, you may not have been taught good dental care and therefore may have gradually lost your teeth. For many people, visits to a dentist were expensive and few and far between, so proper instruction and treatment were never received. If you do not know about proper dental hygiene, it may seem easier and cheaper to have your teeth removed rather than restored. For some, having "artificial" teeth may seem to be a welcome relief from the repairs needed to keep their own.

After the age of twenty-five or thirty, the number of *dental caries* (cavities) decreases, so it is unlikely that you will lose your teeth because of this. As you get older, there is often a thinning and decrease in calcium in the bones in your face and jaw. Along with the loss of bone, the health of your gums may deteriorate. Strong bones and sound gums are needed to support your teeth.

Poor gum care is a common problem. Lack of proper dental hygiene often leads to the formation of debris and calcium deposits (*plaque* and *calculus*) at the base of your teeth. This eventually causes gum inflammation and infection, and eventually they may no longer be able to hold your teeth in place. The end result may be loosening of your teeth and their eventual loss. If you still have some of your own teeth, it is preferable to try and keep them. Sometimes this requires dental restoration (rebuilding) and treatment of the surrounding gums.

Natural teeth form an excellent support for dentures. Even one or two teeth that are stable and firmly implanted in the bones of your mouth can make a good base for partial dentures. Rather than extracting teeth, it is sometimes preferable to grind the remaining teeth down to the surface of the gums and use them for supports. At least some of the missing teeth should be replaced in order to allow proper chewing and digestion of food.

When partial dentures are made, they must be designed for easy removal. Your dentist should take into account any physical disability you may have. A special design may be necessary to permit you to take care of your dentures, especially if you have a handicap such as arthritis. But the most important step in maintaining your dentures is good oral hygiene. You should learn to clean your dentures as well as your own teeth and keep up the condition of your gums. Inflammation and infections should always receive immediate attention.

Occasionally, your gums may become irritated by poorly fitting dentures. This should be treated by removing your dentures until your gums recover. If it recurs, your dentist should examine your dentures and gums. He may be able to modify your dentures so that you can enjoy your food.

As your facial bones vary and the shape of your gums change, it may be necessary to adjust, reline, and alter your dentures. Your dentist should evaluate this if the changes have occurred recently. In many situations where dentures have not fitted properly for many years, it might be almost impossible to repair them or to make new, better-fitting dentures. With well-designed, properly fitting dentures, the use of adhesives is rarely necessary.

Certain precautions should be taken when going for dental care. Remember that your dentist should be informed of all the medications that you are taking. This is especially the case if you are taking sedatives, tranquilizers, or anticoagulants. Major dental surgery should not be done if you are taking anticoagulants because it can cause serious bleeding. It is essential also to remind your dentist of medical problems, such as heart disease, high blood pressure, and diabetes mellitus. Allergies to medications such as painkillers (analgesics) and antibiotics should be put in your dental record.

A most important illness that may affect you if precautions are not taken is *bacterial endocarditis* (see page 276). If you have a heart murmur, you *must* inform your dentist because antibiotic treatment is frequently necessary. It is given just before the dental treatment is begun and continued for forty-eight hours after the work is completed. If he is not sure of the appropriate antibiotic treatment, he should ask your physician before working on your teeth. Overlooking this problem can lead to serious consequences.

NONMEDICAL SPECIALISTS

There are many nonmedical professionals whose care is vitally important for you to maintain an optimum level of health. Like physicians, they require a lengthy education, and depending on the country, many may be called "doctor." It is important to know how best to utilize the services of these specialists. They often work closely with physicians, and frequently you may be referred to one of them by your own physician.

PODIATRISTS AND CHIROPODISTS

The care of your feet is as important as the care of the rest of your body. Although few medical doctors limit their practice to feet alone, *podiatrists* and *chiropodists* are trained to deal with foot problems. Different countries have various requirements for their training and different diplomas are awarded. In some countries certain types of surgery can be done by these specialists, and in others treatment is more confined.

Some people go to these practitioners without a referral from their physician. However, you should tell your physician that you have been to a foot specialist and relate any special problems that were encountered. It is extremely important that you tell every physician or nonphysician if you suffer from diabetes mellitus or peripheral vascular disease. Also, remember to tell the practitioner about the medications that you are taking, especially if they include anticoagulants (blood thinners).

Your feet are your passport to life. Many people ignore foot care, and consequently their ability to enjoy mobility is greatly impaired. Maintaining your independence should be one of your major goals. The ability to walk easily, in comfort, and without assistance is crucial to self-sufficiency. The condition of your feet can make the difference between your being able to manage alone and needing institutional care. Furthermore, the condition of your feet reflects the general state of your health, and it may affect it seriously.

It is common for the elderly to develop toenails that are thick, hard, and difficult to cut. Nail care may be unmanageable if you have poor eyesight or other physical disabilities that interfere with the proper bathing of your feet and cutting of your nails. There are a number of causes of thick toenails, including the aging process itself, repeated injury to the nails, various types of inflammation, and a poor blood supply. Debris often collects under the nails and discolors them and increases their hardness. Infections, especially fungus infections, may compound the problem.

Treatment is usually best supervised by either a podiatrist or chiropodist. Cleaning and removing the debris that collects around the nails and trimming them periodically is very important. Occasionally, your whole nail may have to be removed if it is thick, hard, and misshapen.

Another problem that causes pain and disability is *callus* formation. This area of hardened skin occurs because there is an abnormal amount of pressure on part of your foot, usually from shoes that do not fit properly. The first step in treating a callus is to remove the cause of the pressure. This usually means changing shoes and finding ones that fit correctly. Special inserts and supports can be fitted into shoes to take the pressure off the affected areas.

Treating your calluses by yourself can be dangerous. Cutting them with knives and razor blades is very hazardous. Commercial callus-removing preparations sometimes destroy the surrounding skin and lead to infection. Treatment is best carried out by a foot specialist, who may surgically shave the excessively hardened callus in stages. He will also help you select proper shoes so that the callus will have less stimulation for its return.

To keep your feet in good condition, a number of principles should be followed. It is very important that you have shoes that are properly fitted and correct for the kind of activities you normally do. Narrow-toed shoes should be avoided. Many older women have been used to wearing high-heeled shoes for years. Your legs may be more comfortable in a heel, even in your later years. A low heel is acceptable, especially if the shoes have wide toes. For those with relatively few foot problems, ordinary shoes may be suitable.

Some people with severe foot problems may need to have special shoes made. This is best done under the supervision of a chiropodist, podiatrist, orthopedic surgeon, or physiatrist (rehabilitation expert) in order to avoid unnecessary expense. The shoes should be purchased from a reputable, experienced foot-wear firm, and one that will service your shoes after you purchase them. Sometimes shoes can be modified so that they are easier to put on. For example, laces are often difficult to tie if you have arthritis or poor eyesight, so a Velcro closure can be substituted by a shoemaker.

If your feet are swollen, the fitting of shoes may be difficult. Excess pressure on swollen feet can be dangerous. If you suffer from swollen feet, your physician can recommend treatment. The swelling may be the result of varicose veins or heart failure. Avoid stockings with tight bands at the top which can exaggerate foot swelling.

It is very important to cut your toenails properly. Nails should be cut straight across, and they should not be cut too short. Sometimes it is easier to cut your nails after bathing your feet because the nails will be softer. Wash and dry your feet carefully every day or two, and inspect them for breaks in the skin and reddened areas.

Many older people suffer from a poor blood supply to their feet. If you have diabetes mellitus, this may be even more exaggerated, particularly if you smoke. Infection around nails or between toes is also common, especially following a foot injury or the improper cutting of nails. Infections can be very dangerous if you have a poor blood supply or diabetes mellitus. Seek medical attention immediately if you notice an infection. If not treated properly and effectively, toes and feet can suffer from gangrene, which could result in the loss of a leg.

Never put your feet in very hot or very cold water. The temperature of water should be tested with your hand first. Using electric pads and hot water bottles on your feet is not recommended. You may have a poor sense of temperature, and your feet could be burned without your realizing it.

A common foot disorder that leads to pain and disability is *bunions,* the cause of which is complex. Some people seem to be more prone to this deformity, which eventually leads to a painful protrusion at the side of the big toe. Very narrow shoes worn during your formative years may have aggravated the condition, but some people develop bunions even though they have always worn properly-fitting shoes. At a younger age, surgery is usually recommended for bunions. In most cases it relieves the deformity and improves many of the symptoms of pain and inflammation in the region of the protruding bone. However, as you grow older, the chances of improving the condition with surgery gradually decrease, and the relative risks of foot surgery increase.

If you are otherwise in good health and do not suffer from diabetes mellitus or diseased blood vessels and your bunions are causing great discomfort, ask your physician to refer you to an orthopedic surgeon. For many older people, however, it is probably better to have a special shoe molded to the misshapen foot in order to relieve the pain and irritation rather than undergo surgery.

OPTOMETRISTS AND OPTICIANS

Vision is crucial to our well-being, but there is a great deal of confusion about who is qualified to examine eyes. In most Western countries physicians are trained to evaluate major diseases that may show signs of affecting the eye. If you have diabetes mellitus or high blood pressure, for example, your physician will periodically examine your eyes with an *ophthalmoscope,* which illuminates the retina. The progress of these diseases can sometimes be judged by the condition of the blood vessels in the retina.

For a serious eye condition your physician will usually send you to an *ophthalmologist* (eye specialist). In order to receive his diploma, he must have a further three to five years of training after medical school. Therefore, an ophthalmologist is a medical doctor who can evaluate and treat abnormal conditions of the eye and perform eye surgery.

Many people confuse nonmedical eye specialists who are trained to perform specific services related to vision with ophthalmologists, who *are* physicians. Depending on the country, state, or province, the training of these professionals varies, and what they are permitted to do may differ. An *optician* is primarily responsible for grinding lenses according to a prescription, but he may also be allowed to fit and sell lenses. However, he does not examine eyes.

Optometrists have special training in the visual sciences. Although often titled "doctor," they are nonmedical specialists. They can examine eye movements and test for errors in *refraction* (sharpness of vision), and in many areas they are allowed to test eye pressure. Although trained to recognize major abnormalities of the eye, they have limited knowledge of the many complex eye problems that especially affect the elderly. They may work closely with an optician and thus both examine eyes and sell glasses.

In order to get optimal eye care, you should know which of these professionals to consult. An optometrist may be the first person to suspect that you have an eye disorder if you return frequently to have your glasses changed. A careful eye examination by an optometrist may reveal early signs of glaucoma, cataracts, infections of the eye, or retinal diseases. Because of the many disorders that can affect the eyes of older people— and the interactions with medical illnesses and their treatments—an ophthalmologist should be consulted periodically. If your general health is good and your vision relatively stable, you should see an ophthalmologist once a year. You can expect a full examination of the pressure in your eye, an evaluation that you can see fully in all directions, an assessment of whether you may be developing cataracts, and a full look at your retina. The muscles and other tissues of the eyes will also be examined. If you need a change in glasses, the ophthalmologist can give you a prescription, which can be filled by an optician.

Full cooperation among these professionals is the rule, and you should take advantage of each in their areas of expertise. Although it is a common practice, do not rely exclusively on the services of a nonphysician specialist to care for your eyes. Many senior-citizen centers, outpatient clinics, nursing homes, and homes for the aged make arrangements with all these specialists to have regular eye examinations for their members.

NUTRITIONISTS AND DIETITIANS

Although nutrition is a major industry, physicians have the reputation of "not being interested" in nutrition. This is not quite accurate: Most physicians have the basic knowledge to answer questions on nutrition, but over the years they have not used their education and experience to give nutritional advice. Lately, a greater emphasis and interest on nutritional problems is being taught in medical schools.

Nutritionists and dietitians are nonmedical practitioners who are often consulted by physicians to give advice to patients, particularly regarding diets for weight reduction, high blood pressure, heart or vascular disease, and diabetic control. Many institutions employ them to assist patients and residents in following appropriate diets. Depending on locale, educational requirements differ for dietitians and nutritionists. A dietitian has a bachelor's degree in chemistry and nutrition, often with postgraduate training. In many places, a qualified nutritionist has postgraduate training in addition to a bachelor's degree but, unfortunately, many people who refer to themselves as "nutritionists" have no formal training or certification.

Most Western countries have national and local associations that disseminate information on health and nutrition. They may also monitor and make recommendations to governments or other organizations about such areas as food additives or proper product labeling.

One problem affecting all of us which may become more pronounced during your later years is the attraction to unusual diets. It may become very alluring to follow the recommendations of dietary practitioners who claim that their diets can solve problems of aging, cancer, heart disease, or many of the common illnesses that plague us as we grow older.

Certain professional schools train people to diagnose and treat many common disorders as though they were all diet-related. Although some of the points may be well founded and glowing results are often claimed by people who have followed one of these dietary regimens, many of the principles have not been adequately tested or proven and do not coincide with traditional medical teaching. Similar assertions are often made for the innumerable weight-reduction programs that fill the pages of newspapers, magazines, and the shelves of bookstores and libraries. If the foundation of the diet does not contradict the principles of balance, variety, and calorie control, it is probably not dangerous and possibly may be beneficial, although the benefits may be difficult to determine.

The basic principles of nutrition as commonly accepted and understood by most physicians, dietitians, and qualified nutritionists are discussed in Chapter 4.

CHAPTER 3

The Psychology of Aging

THE NORMAL PSYCHOLOGICAL ASPECTS OF AGING

It is often assumed that as a natural consequence of the aging process people develop severe psychological and memory problems. This belief is so widely held that when an older person is emotionally and intellectually well preserved, one often hears a comment such as, "She's eighty years old and still with it." It seems that everyone believes that as you enter your later years, your mind shuts itself off and you are merely idly waiting to pass from this world.

It may surprise many people, including health care personnel who have not had broad experience with the elderly, that relatively few significant psychological changes are associated with aging. It is unlikely that your personality or memory will change as you age. You will probably be more certain of your beliefs if they have persisted and survived many years, so some people may consider you to be stubborn. Or you may be as flexible and reasonable as you have always been. If you always had a sense of humor, you will still have it, and if the world always seemed dark and dismal, it probably will not improve.

As you grow older, you may experience some changes in your psychological function and mental abilities. These, however, are minimal. If you have always been a stable, highly motivated, interested, and creative person, in all likelihood you will continue to be so as you grow older. Your age should make no difference in the way you look at life. Our emotional makeup does not change as much as we think. Those people who were independent when they were younger will almost invariably try to be so even when they are ill or disabled. On the other hand, those who always sought help and assistance during their younger years will do so even more as they grow older. They may even use the excuse of "growing old" to *get* sympathy and assistance.

Significant changes in your personality, memory, or emotional stability are more likely to come from an illness, either physical or psychological, than from the aging process itself. Therefore, it is important, when you or your family notice such changes, that a thorough investigation be done to determine the underlying cause so that appropriate treatment can be recommended.

One often hears the word *senility* used to describe the process by which older people seem to lose their memory and become mentally confused. The word is used too freely and loosely. Senility, in fact, means *getting old*. The word has nothing to do with memory or personality. Because it is often applied uncritically to people with emotional or memory difficulties, a more objective assessment may never be seriously pursued.

Only a small proportion of the elderly suffer serious memory loss as they age. The term *dementia* is used to describe the different kinds of memory impairment that affect *some* older individuals. You may find some difficulty learning complex, new information, but you may not be as *interested* in learning new information if you think it has little value to you. But this is not so much a difficulty in memory as much as a lack of motivation.

For example, an older couple came to see me because the wife was concerned that her husband was losing his memory. He did not agree with her, but after much coaxing he agreed to visit my office. They seemed to have had a very long and generally satisfying marriage. She was an avid bridge enthusiast, and over the years he had learned the game and joined her in playing, but never with any great relish. She now complained that he constantly made mistakes and "forgot" how to play the game.

During the interview I did not detect any significant impairment of the husband's memory or learning abilities. He was well informed in current events, could discuss recent books he had read, and was able to deal with complex mental problems. When I went into the examining room to evaluate him, he told me quietly, "I so dislike bridge that I just am not interested in playing." His problem was a lack of motivation rather than a loss of memory. In addition, he did not want to disappoint his wife, who depended on his playing bridge with her. Rather than telling her that he would rather not play, he played badly. I discussed this with his wife, and she agreed to make fewer demands on him for bridge engagements, and he agreed to try and play as well as he could during the games that he would attend.

An effective memory depends on many factors. You must concentrate on the subject in order to remember it. Your brain has to absorb the information and then store it for a later date. You should be able to put ideas and memories into a language that is clear and meaningful to you and to others. If any part of this memory circuit is impaired or damaged, you will not be able to communicate those ideas and memories.

If indeed you begin to find that your memory is failing, or if your family notices that you are forgetting things and becoming confused, a thorough investigation should be made. It is mandatory to look for possible causes of memory loss that are treatable or reversible. No one should assume that the loss of memory is the result of age alone.

One of the disorders that can cause memory loss and which may improve with treatment is *hypothyroidism* (underactive thyroid gland). A lack of *vitamin B12* or *folic acid* can also cause memory impairment, even without the anemia that usually occurs with this deficiency.

Sometimes a *brain tumor* or a disturbance called *normotensive hydrocephalus* can appear as memory loss. These disorders can usually be diagnosed by a careful neurological (nervous system) investigation. In some cases surgery may relieve the condition, and an improvement in memory may follow.

A common cause of memory loss and mental confusion is the *cumulative effects of medications*. Some drugs, such as tranquilizers and sleeping pills, cause this more than others. However, certain medications used to treat high blood pressure, heart disease, Parkinson's disease, allergies, or pain can also cause this. Because of the many drug benefit programs for the elderly (such as Medicare), you may accidentally be taking more than one drug of the same type without realizing it. This is because similar medications may be prescribed that have different names. This problem is compounded if you do not use the same pharmacist for all your prescriptions.

Another important and frequently overlooked cause of memory impairment is *depression*. You may not feel the usual symptoms of this disorder, and you, your family, and your physician may not even consider this as the cause of your impediment. It is quite common to be labeled senile because of depression. As the illness progresses, you may forget what is happening around you and emotionally and mentally withdraw from the world (see page 56).

Unfortunately, some causes of memory loss and changes in personality are not reversible. But this does not mean that certain aspects of the condition cannot be improved. For instance, agitated and frustrated behavior can be controlled. This is sometimes accomplished by modifying living arrangements and activities, or through judicious use of drug therapy.

One frequent cause of memory impairment and mental confusion for which there is no cure is *Alzhemier's disease*. A great deal of research is being done to try to discover the basis for this illness so that an effective therapy can be found. The disorder results in a gradual and progressive loss of brain cells, which manifests itself in persistent and continued loss of memory and judgment. Alteration in personality, with episodes of aggressive or agitated behavior, can make it difficult to receive proper attention. Some of these symptoms can be controlled or modified. When aggressive or violent behavior occurs, small doses of tranquilizers may produce a calming effect.

Among the most important methods of treatment for Alzheimer's disease is provision of an environment that will allow the individual to move and act as freely as possible without danger to himself or other people. This may require that activities be organized in which the person can participate at a level that is suitable and not frustrating. Dissipation of energy in physical activities such as walking and dancing can be very beneficial. Unfortunately, people with this illness are often put into institutions and given excessive amounts of tranquilizers so that they will not bother the nursing and medical staff. People treated this way often end up sleeping most of the time, and they become mentally and physically inactive or even bedridden.

Enlightened institutions have learned that most people afflicted with this disorder respond to stimulation and reminders of what is going on in the world. In most instances, although *recent* memory may become impaired, recollection of past events will remain quite good. Therefore, emphasis should be put on things that have happened many years ago. The person should be encouraged to talk about past experiences and urged to become involved in social activities. Since it may be difficult to judge the quality of institutional care, the family may have to take responsibility for assuring appropriate treatment. This can be done by speaking to the administrative, nursing and social service staff to determine what programs are planned and what the philosophy of the institution is regarding this type of problem. Sometimes, several families that are willing to work together can stimulate the organization to develop a volunteer service that will develop programs to keep mentally impaired older patients suitably occupied.

Another cause of memory difficulties is *atherosclerosis* of the blood vessels going to and located in the brain, which may result in a number of small "strokes." This can also make movement and speech difficult. Usually the disease is less gradual than Alzheimer's disease, and it occurs in episodes. Some improvement may be seen between each small stroke, but ultimately the damage may be severe and memory loss great.

Over the years, many drugs have been developed that are claimed to reverse memory loss. Since memory impairment has many different causes, it can be hard to determine whether or not a particular medication is effective. If a specific cause for memory loss is found, then a specific drug such as thyroid hormone or antidepressants may be effective.

If no specific treatable cause for memory loss is found, some families unfortunately seek unconventional treatments that claim to be successful. These include "special" vitamins and unusual drugs. Often, a great deal of counseling is required before family members accept that no completely satisfactory treatment or miraculous cures exist. Before it is assumed that there is no reversible cause for memory loss, your physician should investigate those illnesses for which there is treatment. This may also save a family from frantically looking for nonexistent cures and from becoming victims of charlatans or drug distributors that use such feelings of desperation to sell their products.

In the past few years a number of naturally occurring substances have been studied that seem to have important effects on the brain. It has been shown that some of the important nervous system functions involved in memory depend on substances that are influenced by the amount of *choline* in the diet. Several preliminary studies suggest that in certain neurological disorders and some types of memory loss, supplementation with large doses of choline may be effective. Other studies show that *lecithin* is changed into choline, and the same effects can be achieved with fewer side effects. The results of a number of controlled preliminary studies using these substances for treatment of Alzheimer's disease have, however, been less encouraging than originally hoped.

What does this mean to the ordinary older person? Should you take large supplemental doses of choline, which can cause nausea, or lecithin, which is quite expensive, in order to *prevent* the possibility of memory loss? There is no conclusive evidence to show that if you take these substances while you are well and have a good memory, this enviable state will be maintained or improved.

However, for those people who are experiencing the first signs of Alzheimer's disease or other types of progressive memory loss, these substances could be added to the diet. However, you should use them only under the supervision of your physician or a neurologist. The cost of these substances is considerable, and to take them unnecessarily can be a waste of money and a disappointing experience. In addition, other important, treatable causes of memory loss may be missed if you rely on self-medication without consulting your physician.

ANXIETY AND THE USE OF TRANQUILIZERS

It would be foolish and unrealistic to believe that there are no emotional difficulties associated with aging. That younger people often need psychological treatment and counseling is a reflection of a real human necessity that does not stop with age. In many ways your psychological makeup will change very little over the years. If you have had few psychological problems, you will probably continue to be stable in your mature years. If you have had many problems in coping with the stresses of life, this will probably continue as you age. Of course, even the most stable, well-balanced older person may experience new challenges and unanticipated difficulties that will affect his or her psychological balance. Unexpected tragedies have a deep influence on our emotional well-being.

All of us at some time have experienced *anxiety*. It is an uncomfortable and sometimes terrifying experience. You may feel your heart racing, your head thumping, and your palms perspiring. You may lose your appetite or overeat. You may feel like pacing the floor, and you may experience fitful sleeping. The feeling may come and go throughout the day or last for weeks or months. In most instances there is usually an easily identifiable cause for your anxiety. Perhaps someone you love is severely ill. Perhaps you are in the midst of a major financial crisis, or a disaster has befallen your home or family. At other times, the event precipitating an attack of anxiety may be less severe. You may have had last-minute changes in travel arrangements, or you may have been in an automobile accident and you or your family almost injured. You may be waiting for a phone call from a loved one, and it is delayed and you do not know why. There are countless causes of this type of anxiety. In most instances, once the situation causing the anxious feeling is resolved, the emotional strain disappears and the symptoms go away.

Some people seem to worry constantly. It may be a lifelong pattern and have little to do with major new challenges or dangers. I know older women who constantly and chronically worry about the welfare of their children. If you look back at their earlier experiences, they may have been overbearing mothers. Even though their children may be grown and independent, these mothers may become anxious if they do not receive frequent phone calls to confirm that their children are well.

Some people seem to be anxious about everything in general and nothing in particular. When they hear a news broadcast, they worry. When they read a newspaper, they fret. They do not seem to be geared for the natural and unavoidable consequences of living. Sometimes their anxiety can be so great that they become immobilized.

Many medications have been developed during the past decades that have a major effect on the symptoms and feelings associated with anxiety. Because they calm the emotions, the medications are called *tranquilizers.* Of the various types, some are effective for milder degrees of anxiety, while others are used for more serious emotional disturbances. Many years ago, *barbiturates* were frequently used as tranquilizers. These drugs accumulate in the body and can have many serious side effects. They are rarely, if ever, used for this purpose in older individuals, and they should *never* be used for emotional disorders.

One group of drugs, referred to as minor tranquilizers, include *diazepam* and *chlordiazepoxide,* which are sold under many brand names, including the popular Valium® and Librium®. There is a great deal of controversy as to whether these drugs have any place in the treatment of emotional disorders in the older population, however.

As is often the case with many medications, it may take years before the full benefits and unwanted side effects of tranquilizers are known. There is no question that they decrease feelings of anxiety and reduce or abolish the uncomfortable symptoms. However, they do not in any way deal with the underlying cause of the disorder. Tranquilizers cannot alter the outside world; If you are anxious because you think your well-being is threatened, they will numb your feelings for awhile, but they will not alter the reality of your situation. However, sometimes the degree of anxiety is greatly out of proportion to the real events causing it. A minor tranquilizer can calm you until you can evaluate more realistically just what has happened to make you anxious. For these purposes, tranquilizers probably have value.

These drugs have caused concern in their use among the elderly because often they are overused, and in quantities that may be cumulative and harmful. It was believed for a long time that they had few side effects, so less care was taken in their use. Some older people tend to accumulate these medications in their bodies, because of decreased ability to metabolize them, with resultant serious side effects. But the most disturbing consequence of their use is dulling of the mind and mental confusion.

Another serious consequence is overlooking a medical condition that may require a specific kind of treatment, or the exaggeration of a depressive illness, which may be aggravated by these drugs. They may also interact with other preparations that act on the mind, such as antihistamines, anti-parkinsonism medications, hypertension drugs and sleeping pills. A combination of drugs may make it appear that you are losing your memory.

In general, minor tranquilizers should be used sparingly and infrequently. If you have been using them for many years, you should try to find out why you require them by consulting your physician or a psychological counselor. If you occasionally become anxious and know that a small dose helps you, it is probably acceptable to use them.

If you notice that you require increasing amounts of these drugs, however, consult your physician to see if there is another disorder that may be exaggerating your problems. Do not increase the dosage on your own. It is amazing how many people, including the elderly, become dependent on tranquilizers and are often afraid to discontinue them. It is always worthwhile to try to decrease them. It may take a few weeks to do so as you gradually limit the amount you take. Many people have been able to stop taking them altogether, even after using them for many years.

Since your emotional condition is usually a reflection of your personality, any major change in your feelings or behavior should be carefully examined. Most people do not think of themselves as "old" until they experience a severe illness or a condition that limits their ability to function fully and actively. If this happens, you may suddenly feel an enormous emotional strain, perhaps as a result of loneliness, isolation, or loss of a loved one. In addition, financial, social, and physical difficulties may occur with aging, and these may increase your anxiety. In many instances a proper examination and full evaluation of your emotional and social condition can lead to beneficial recommendations. And a properly directed program of treatment may return you to a fuller, more satisfying life.

DEPRESSION AND OTHER EMOTIONAL DISORDERS

Many people use the word *depression* when they really mean unhappiness or disappointment. Unlike the younger person, you may find it hard to admit that you are depressed. You may feel that your lack of positive feelings and motivation is part of the aging process. You may lose interest in things that you formerly enjoyed and become overly concerned with your physical health. Eventually, your family and physician may ignore your laments, and this often worsens your condition as your cry for help goes unheeded.

Depression may be easily overlooked as you grow older. You may lose your appetite and lose weight, which may make you or your physician think of a physical illness such as cancer. This only adds to your feelings of desperation. If you have difficulty sleeping, you may ask for tranquilizers and sleeping pills, which could aggravate your symptoms. You may also have feelings of guilt about your family. When things become very bad, you may begin to lose your sense of self-worth.

Depression is one of the most prevalent illnesses that affects the older generation. Because often it is not recognized, many people do not receive proper therapy. Younger family members may assume that it is "normal" for you to become depressed as you age and not recognize your symptoms as being caused by an illness that, like many physical ailments, can be treated successfully.

Often there is a precipitating cause for a depressive illness. It could be an emotional trauma, such as the death of a spouse or a child. At other times, it may be a physical illness, such as a heart attack, stroke, or pneumonia. In these instances, although you may make a good physical recovery, you may feel that you have not returned to your "old self." This may be the first sign of a depressive illness.

The grandmother of one of my colleagues was admitted to the hospital because of a lung infection. She had severe pneumonia and required many days of intensive antibiotic therapy before she was out of danger. Prior to becoming ill, she lived on her own, close to her family, and managed well. Despite our high expectations, she did not recuperate quickly, and she began to spend more time in bed, despite the urging of her family and the medical staff that she should start becoming more active.

She finally reached a point where she lay in bed all day, curled up like a baby. She stopped eating. When put in a chair, she would look ahead and respond to questions with one or two words. After ten days of antidepressive medication, she brightened up and within a few weeks was able to return home, back to her usual activity and interest in life. Hers was an example of depression that was brought on by an illness, in this case pneumonia.

Depression can not only be dangerous but also possibly fatal. If you give up the will to live, it may go so far as to end up with an attempt at suicide. Unfortunately, this is common in older persons. It seems to affect men more often than women because men appear to cope less well with loneliness and isolation. When they become depressed, they often become despondent, completely withdrawing from friends and family. Some people stop eating altogether and become bedridden. Others become institutionalized and labeled "senile."

Despite common beliefs, depression is treatable. Your physician may refer you to a psychiatrist, or he may treat you himself. Your physician can help you examine your social and physical environment to ensure that as many positive factors as possible can be arranged to help support you during your depression. Visits from friends and relatives may help dispel some of your feelings of loneliness and isolation. Assistance from psychiatrists, social workers, nurses, and other community workers may be very helpful. In many communities, volunteer visitors are available. Persistent encouragement and positive attitudes may tide you over an exceptionally difficult period in your life.

The new antidepressant medications are frequently effective. They should be started in very small doses for a period of seven to ten days. This allows time to evaluate both the negative effects and the positive effects. The dose may then be increased. The medication works gradually, and you should not expect to feel better immediately. When you do improve, a maintenance dose is continued for a number of months. Sometimes it can be stopped then, or you may require small doses for a longer period.

Antidepressant medication may be given as a single dose at bedtime. Some people become drowsy at first, and during the first few days you might feel dizzy or tired in the morning. It is very important that you continue the medication, however. This side effect usually wears off within a few days. After two or three weeks you should begin to feel better, and your friends and family may notice a marked improvement in your appearance and activity.

In some severely depressed older people, drug therapy may not be effective, so consultation with a psychiatrist is highly recommended. Sometimes hospitalization and *electroconvulsive therapy* (shock treatment) can have a positive therapeutic effect. This treatment should only be recommended if you have become so severely depressed that your health and life are in jeopardy and if you have not responded to or tolerated conventional antidepressant drug therapy. Although not used commonly, when employed for the treatment of extremely depressed people, its effect can be dramatic. Patients who have entered a state of complete withdrawal, refusing to eat or communicate, have responded to such therapy within a matter of a few days or weeks.

After electroconvulsive therapy, there may be a period of temporary mental confusion which usually disappears in time. Because of the negative feelings associated with this treatment, many people fear it and consequently refuse it even though it might be extremely beneficial.

Although drugs used to treat emotional problems can be beneficial, they are not without possible side effects. One major hazard is using sedatives and tranquilizers to treat insomnia and "nervousness," rather than treating the underlying depressive illness. Another problem is that a dosage suitable for a younger person may be excessive for the older person. You may experience dizziness, drowsiness, and an uncomfortable dryness in your mouth if you receive too large a dose. Because of these side effects, you may refuse to continue the medication.

Even with the proper dose, you may feel some drowsiness for the first few days. Therefore, the drug should be taken at night. If the medication causes confusion at first, a smaller dose should be tried. A dry mouth may be an unavoidable consequence, however, and trouble with urination can also occur.

Another problem is that some people who feel suicidal may not be active enough to carry out their wish to die, but when they receive antidepressants, there may be a short period when they still feel depressed, and they may be sufficiently active to succeed. Although this is very uncommon, it is important to have proper supervision from family or professionals, especially early in therapy. Some people with severe heart disease may not be able to tolerate antidepressants. However, in small doses, most can benefit from the newer drugs, which affect the heart less severely than the older ones.

Severe depression that goes unrecognized can lead to memory impairment, which often is mislabeled as senility. You may stop communicating and appear to have severe memory loss. Some individuals may develop incontinence of urine and bowels, and total nursing care may be required. Some people with this condition are inappropriately institutionalized because the depressive illness is not recognized. If you develop relatively sudden memory loss, and if you have had recent emotional or physical stress, you may be suffering from *pseudodementia* which is due to depression. In many instances antidepressant medication markedly improves your memory and function.

Sometimes depression alternates with feelings of great euphoria. In most instances this type of behavior can be traced back to earlier years, when it may have been overlooked. This can be the sign of a *manic-depressive* illness. During the periods of euphoria, or mania, people lose some of their critical abilities and suffer impaired judgment. They may make promises that they cannot keep or invest or spend money foolishly. They may become overactive and have difficulty sleeping. Sometimes it is thought that they just have too much energy. The period of mania may be followed by a stage of severe depression and despondency. This condition can be treated successfully in most instances. The drug *lithium* is often effective in preventing the periods of mania, and this alone may be sufficient to control the disorder, including the bouts of depression. Sometimes small doses of antidepressant medications are also useful.

Although depression is the most common psychological problem in older people, any other psychological illness that you may have suffered from previously may continue into your later years. There are older people who have been *schizophrenics* throughout their adult lives. Their symptoms may be less severe as they grow older, but under certain circumstances, they also may increase.

Some older people become *paranoid*, although, like schizophrenia, often they had this type of personality throughout their lives. They are suspicious and frequently isolate themselves from others because they are afraid that people are attacking them both physically and psychologically, and they may even call the police for help against their imaginary enemies. For the most part these psychological problems can be managed with appropriate changes in the environment. At times, small doses of medications may be necessary to decrease the symptoms and allow the older person to remain at home, rather than being institutionalized.

Sometimes an older individual who is relatively well and functioning independently suddenly becomes mentally confused. The actual cause of the *confusion* may be mistakenly diagnosed as senility and the underlying reason overlooked entirely. The more suddenly that one's memory becomes impaired, the more likely that it is the result of a physical or emotional problem that can be treated and reversed. A physical illness such as an infection, heart attack, or an overfilled urinary bladder may also cause mental confusion. Following surgery, you may become confused because of the anesthetic or medications that are used to treat pain and nausea. Many prescription or over-the-counter drugs also can cause confusion. Simply discontinuing the medications may result in a remarkable improvement in mental function.

If you experience sudden memory impairment or mental confusion, consult your physician for a complete examination of all aspects of your physical and emotional condition. He should search for those causes that can be reversed. Never accept a diagnosis of senility without a full investigation. If necessary, get another opinion.

An excellent example concerns a lady in her early seventies who was brought to a hospital emergency room by her husband because she was pacing around the house and seemed to be forgetful. They had moved a few weeks before from their family home, where they had lived for almost forty years and where they had raised their children. A week after the move, the husband noticed that his wife had been sleeping poorly, talking a great deal about her children, and gradually becoming disorganized and disoriented. The physician in the emergency room inadvertently diagnosed her memory impairment as a "sign of senility" and recommended that the husband find an institutional living arrangement for his wife.

Following a reexamination in my office, it became clear that this woman's confusion was precipitated by an emotionally trying move from her own home to a new apartment. She expressed guilt about having abandoned her home and talked about being worthless now that she was "so old." She was admitted to the psychiatry department, where it was confirmed that she was experiencing a depressive illness, accompanied by a great deal of anxiety and agitation. She was treated successfully over the following six weeks with antidepressant medication. After she was discharged from the hospital, she returned home and baked cookies for the entire medical staff. It would have been tragic if the diagnosis of senility had not been questioned.

DEATH AND DYING

We all must die sooner or later. Those of us who are fortunate die only after a long, healthy, productive life. Some of us die after a prolonged illness, and some die suddenly without warning. We often hear people say that it is best to die "suddenly and painlessly." Of course, such a death deprives us of the opportunity of saying our final words to loved ones and making preparations that will be important to the family. Most of us would agree, however, that a long and painful death would not be welcome. On the other hand, many illnesses are prolonged. Most people have a very strong desire to live, and this tenacity for life must be respected by families and the medical profession.

The question of whether or not treatment should be given to prolong the life of an older individual raises many moral, ethical, and medical problems. Many people assume that as you get older death seems less frightening and more attractive.

This is usually not so. Most of us at every age continue to have the curiosity and interest that make us want to live.

The problem of wanting to die is usually promoted by pain and suffering rather than by age. No one welcomes discomfort and disability. It is often difficult for children and members of the medical profession to ignore a sick older person's request to be "allowed to die." Before a decision to treat certain problems is made, it is important to decide what the likely outcome will be. Success must also be judged in terms of the comfort that will be experienced after therapy. It is all too easy to allow older people to die. On the other hand, heroic measures for which there is little chance of success are not appropriate.

I often meet families who strongly resist telling their loved one of impending death. But each of us should be allowed to take care of our own lives. Whether or not your illness is terminal, you should still be allowed to make your own decisions. Your spouse and children may try to protect you from the emotional strain of confronting death. However, you are probably much stronger than your family thinks you are. You should make your plans and then discuss them with family and friends.

Most of us would probably prefer to be told gently and appropriately. Your family should consult your physician so that what is being said to you is consistent. Nobody likes to hear conflicting explanations. You should make time to share your thoughts, fears, and wishes with your family. Warm physical contact is important from the medical and nursing personnel and especially from members of your family. Showing affection and love through stroking, hugging, and touching are very soothing, so never be afraid to give it and ask for it in return.

Pain and other forms of discomfort should be treated as effectively as possible. Some effective pain relievers may cause you to become sleepy, though. You and your family should decide on the relative merits of physical discomfort and mental alertness. If you would prefer to suffer a little more pain in order to remain awake, tell your family and physician so that the dosage of drugs will be tailored to your needs. All too often one sees the family complaining that their loved one is in great pain, and then soon afterward they wonder why the person is so drowsy. A reasonable balance can almost always be found.

Many aspects to your remaining days can be improved. If you have difficulty eating, a nutritionist or dietitian can be helpful in finding foods that are attractive and palatable. Medications can help to decrease nausea and vomiting. There is generally little merit to following restrictive diets when one has few days or weeks of life left. I have often told families to bring in whatever home-cooked delicacies the family member might enjoy, rather than have him turn away one hospital tray after another.

We all want to die in a dignified and private manner. Communication with your spouse and children is very important. You and your family should, as early as possible, make an arrangement with the nursing and medical personnel looking after you as to how problems might be solved. This can be difficult at times in large institutions, but usually a social worker or nursing supervisor can find a suitable solution.

Your family should agree to have one person act as a mutual spokesman so that unnecessary repetition of questions is avoided. Periodic meetings with nursing and medical staff can relieve fear and anxiety. Your family should not be afraid to approach the staff for help.

The process of dying is not easy, but families and health professionals can cooperate to ease the loneliness and pain experienced by those of us who are living our last days.

CHAPTER 4

Living the Good Life

One widely accepted definition of health is that it is the absence of disease. Illness sometimes affects people for no apparent reason, but the more positive your view of life, the less likely you are to succumb to many of the problems that afflict the elderly. A combination of good health habits, sensible nutritional practices, and outlets for physical and emotional energies will go a long way in helping you enjoy healthy and satisfying senior years. And many older individuals seem to have maintained the vigor and spirit to help overcome any physical disabilities. Although physicians may be able to guide you about many aspects of your health care, the principles of living the good life must not only be understood, but must be adopted.

WORK

One reason that people sometimes become physically and emotionally dependent in their later years is because they have left the work force after a long career. Self-esteem and independence are difficult to maintain when you no longer feel that you are making a contribution to society. In addition, families often become fragmented and are geographically separated. This means that you cannot even count on your role as a respected elder, which used to be the case when families remained together. Some professionals can pursue their vocation into their later years, and this allows them to continue being productive and dynamic. However, many people do not have the opportunity to continue working after the age of 65 or 70 because most industries have a retirement age. Some older people fare very well after they retire; many, however, find that time becomes their enemy. The inactivity that frequently follows retirement often leads to excessive preoccupation with the body and concerns about health. Those who find productive and creative outlets for their retirement years seem to have the best chance of maintaining their health and vigor.

Ideally, preparation for this stage of your life should be done long before your actual retirement. But if you have not prepared, new skills and interests can still be developed after you stop working. Hobbies should be pursued to the point where they can satisfactorily fill a good deal of your time. In order to promote your continued involvement with other working and productive people, you can even embark on a new career. Many businesses and stores might welcome your assistance in various tasks. The amount of money that you earn should not be a major consideration. It may even be possible for you to return to your previous place of work with an agreement that you earn a limited income for a limited amount of work. Many employers might welcome the experience and expertise that you can contribute to younger workers.

Look into schools and recreational facilities. For example, you could teach children carpentry, cooking, sewing, bookkeeping, or other useful skills. Hospitals and nursing homes might welcome you as a volunteer to help patients and residents. Remuneration for these activities is less important than the satisfaction that is achieved from productive work and being in touch with others.

I know a woman who is almost 85 years old and who works every day as a volunteer in a home for the aged. She wears her volunteer gown proudly and shows off her pin that she was awarded after she had finished more than 10,000 hours of volunteer work. During the preceding ten years she worked as an assistant to nurses in helping disabled residents in the home with their meals. Whenever she sees me, she comments how she loves helping the "old folks" and does not have time to talk because she is so busy. Her strength and positive outlook have been reinforced by the knowledge that the residents rely on her for their welfare.

Professional people and executives can often find outlets for their skills and training more easily. Many volunteer programs allow skilled older people to act as advisers and instructors. Occasionally, this may require travel, but often positions can be found locally. Even a few days a week or a few hours a day are sufficient to provide incentive and satisfaction.

Some schools and other institutions use the expertise of retired professionals and craftsmen to teach courses. One man I met, who was retiring from his position as a senior baker for a large baking firm, volunteered a few hours a week to teach skills to students of baking and nutrition. He looked forward to his new role in life with great enthusiasm.

RECREATION

As you grow older, you probably will begin to "look forward" to your later years so that you can enjoy the activities that you never had time for before. Then, suddenly you find yourself retired, and time begins to weigh heavily on your hands. If you are a housewife, you may now find that the presence of your husband for many hours a day is difficult to tolerate. He, on the other hand, may find that less time is actually necessary to do the things he always wanted to do, and much of the day seems empty and purposeless. You should reach an agreement with your spouse and children as to how much time each of you can spend with the other comfortably.

Many programs and books are available to help you find an appropriate hobby or activity where you can use your skills. Volunteer or other work can often be combined with hobbies, such as teaching others how to care for plants in a greenhouse club or repair small appliances. You might renew your interest in reading and music, and many clubs in libraries, schools, and senior-citizen centers promote such involvement. Many universities and colleges welcome senior students, and teachers are invariably impressed with the dedication and capabilities of the older student. Going back to school in your later years can be an exciting experience. Your years of practical wisdom become an important asset to your new academic interests.

The retirement years are also a good time to get involved in collecting. Stamps, coins, magazines, antiques, old books, and innumerable other items can be collected. You will have time to go over the items, read about them, and learn their history and meaning. The items do not have to be valuable or even expensive. It is more important that you find something that can maintain your interest.

Some older people decide to raise pets. There may now be time to breed them and even teach other people the skill or start a small business. Animals are a source of satisfaction and company. Many books are written on the subject, and you may be able to get some hints from local pet shops, veterinarians, and even the local zoological society or university.

Gardening is a popular outlet for many older people. Depending on where you live, it may be possible to raise plants outdoors, or you may have to develop a small greenhouse or restrict your skills to plants that can be grown in your home. Plants and flowers can give joy and satisfaction, especially if for some reason you are restricted to your home. You can learn how to grow them for your own pleasure, but you will probably find that many of your neighbors and friends will want to share in your expertise.

The older person who has recreational outlets is usually more productive and satisfied than one who just "sits out" the later years. Many community and senior-citizen centers have excellent programs, and they can be used effectively and positively to supply not only recreation but social activity and friendship. Visit them and give them a try. No doubt you will find fulfillment and satisfaction in whatever hobby or activity you choose.

EXERCISE

Many older people have had little opportunity to be active physically during their adult years. Even if you were athletic in your youth, you probably developed the typical sedentary lifestyle that is so common in our society. Most men get into the habit of driving to work or relying on public transportation to wisk them from their homes to their offices and back again, where they continue with the common activities of television-watching and light household chores. Women are often more active if they have been at home for many years, because raising children and housekeeping require more physical effort than working in an office. Many women, however, have entered the work force and have assumed the same work patterns and activities as men.

What is the result of this gradual decrease in exercise that occurs as you grow older? Weight gain is a common problem. You may find it more and more difficult to maintain your weight, despite heroic attempts at many of the popular diets that abound. Some people may constantly lose weight only to find that the scales catch up with them again a few weeks later.

If your life has been sedentary, you will probably find that even small amounts of physical activity leave you huffing and puffing. A run for a bus or a ball game with a grandchild may completely exhaust you. A long-awaited holiday may prove to be too tiring when you try to explore a new city. You may choose instead to sit out the tour in a fancy tourist bus and never get to feel the enchantment of the place.

No doubt there are many benefits to being physically active as you grow older, including an improvement in the function of your heart, blood vessels, lungs, muscles, and joints. The secret to success is to exercise throughout your life, but if you have not, it is still not too late to get back into good physical shape. And a well-exercised body will feel and look better, thereby improving your emotional well-being.

There are many ways to go about regaining your body tone. If you have not been used to physical activity, you should consult your physician before embarking on an exercise program. He will examine your heart, blood pressure, and lungs, and if you have any problem, he can modify a program to suit you. There is almost never a reason that will prohibit exercise altogether. But beware of commercial "fitness" centers; many of them have little supervision and may not have the means to assess you adequately or design a suitable program. Many senior-citizen centers, schools and YM/WCAs, however, have many well-supervised programs that you can join.

A well-structured agenda will gradually introduce you to various forms of exercise, including walking and slow jogging as well as muscle-loosening calisthenics. The extent and degree of effort will have to be tailored to your own particular health needs. The secret to success is to increase your physical demands gradually and stop when you feel excessively short of breath or fatigued. After many years of being sedentary, do not expect to become an olympic champion overnight. However, continue to increase your efforts gradually in order to achieve your goals.

Certain physical activities generate adequate amounts of exercise and are usually suitable for older persons. *Walking briskly,* in a nice neighborhood or in the country, is an excellent and invigorating form of exercise. If you can do it with a partner, all the better. A slow jog can be added, but this is not necessary for good results.

Bicycle riding is good exercise, but do not take it up unless you were once experienced at it. If you have back trouble, it may not be suitable for you. It is true that you never forget how to ride, but bicycles have changed, and if you are out of practice, go back to it slowly. It should be done easily and gradually. You do not have to race up hills to benefit from cycling. Again, if possible, do it with a partner.

Swimming benefits all the muscles and can be done at a varying pace and with different strokes. It is often combined these days with other activities, such as sitting in a sauna or whirlpool. These can add a certain amount of companionship and invigoration to the swim. Avoid overstaying in the sauna. The benefits of excessive heat and perspiration have not been determined, and it may be dangerous, especially if you have a heart condition or take various medications. Check first with your doctor.

Any activity that combines exercise and social interaction is likely to be beneficial. *Golf* is a fine way of walking and keeping up your sense of companionship and involvement. *Dancing* is a superb form of exercise that is becoming more popular among older people. Many centers offer lessons in all types of dance, and even if you have never danced before, there is a good chance that you can learn fairly easily. The social benefits of dancing are very important and can add a great deal of flavor and spice to your exercise program.

Some types of exercise can be potentially dangerous, especially if you have medical problems. In general, avoid activities that demand sudden bursts of energy. Unless you have always been active in competitive forms of exercise, there is little to be achieved by taking up a sport like tennis. Straining, as in weight lifting, should also be avoided because it puts an excess amount of stress on your heart and blood pressure as well as your back. Even after you have become a seasoned jogger,

71

there may still be a potential danger if you suddenly start sprinting. Take it easy and pace yourself. You will benefit most from your new sense of well-being that follows.

NUTRITION

Good nutrition is essential for health—growth, development, energy, and good body function. We eat for many reasons other than to satisfy nutritional requirements, and most of us have developed eating habits that reflect our social and emotional needs. Because so much of why and what we eat has little to do with our nutritional needs, many of us suffer from poor eating habits and inadequate diets.

Food is divided into *carbohydrates* (sugars and starches), *proteins* (meat, poultry, and fish), and *fats* (from animal and vegetable sources). In addition, many other substances are found in foods, including vitamins and minerals. These help your metabolism and are as important as carbohydrates, proteins, and fats.

Unfortunately, many older people suffer from malnutrition, and this is not limited to the poor and indigent. In fact, many financially secure older people are poorly nourished, as are many younger people. Poor eating habits as much as the unavailability of food or limited funds account for poor nutrition.

As you grow older, your nutritional requirements for growth decrease, but you continue to need nutrients for body maintenance and repair. The only things that you *may* need less of are calories. But although you need smaller amounts of food, you still need a well-balanced diet.

A BALANCED DIET

The key to good nutrition is a balanced diet that contains an adequate amount of calories to maintain your ideal weight and enough of the essential nutrients to keep your body running efficiently. You may need some assistance from your physician or a dietitian to help you decide on a diet to suit you.

A balanced diet should contain carbohydrates, proteins, and fats. The source of *carbohydrate* should contain as little refined sugar as possible. Carbohydrates such as those found in breads, cereals, beans, and vegetables are preferable to those found in sugars and candies. Even though honey may be more flavorful than sugar, it is a simple carbohydrate and therefore less desirable than the other forms of carbohydrate. Small amounts of honey, however, are fine, so long as it is not used instead of other types of carbohydrates.

Proteins are primarily found in meat, fish, and poultry. It is probably best to diversify the type of protein source so that less red meat is eaten and more chicken and fish are substituted. Also, the fat content of red meat is higher than that of poultry and fish. *Vegetable proteins* are available in nuts and legumes (beans and peas), and these should be added to your diet along with other protein sources. Dairy products are an important source of protein as well as calcium. Dairy products play a significant role in maintaining a balanced and varied intake of protein. Eggs, which supply protein as well as fats and vitamins, can be eaten in moderation, from three to four a week.

There has been considerable controversy over the effects of various kinds of fats on health. Much of the data is conflicting and new information appears frequently which seems to change the basis for dietary recommendations. During the past several years, emphasis was placed on decreasing the amount of animal fat in the diet and replacing it with vegetable fats, especially unsaturated varieties.

More recently, however, the basis for these recommendations has come into question. At present it would appear prudent to decrease the amount of animal fat in the diet, primarily in order to maintain your ideal weight. There should be a balance between animal fats—found in dairy products and meat—and vegetable fats and oils, especially the unsaturated type. Some researchers feel that a good part of the vegetable fats should contain *linoleic acid* which is found, for instance, in sunflower-seed oil. Other unsaturated vegetable oils, such as safflower, corn, and soybean, appear to be preferable to saturated varieties such as coconut oil.

The use of margarine is also controversial because the industrial process necessary to solidify the oil may nullify its potential beneficial effect and make it less desirable than previously thought. Some authorities in the field have even gone so far as to recommend increasing the amount of butter in the diet and decreasing the amount of margarine. The answer is probably somewhere in the middle, with a balance between judicious use of animal and vegetable fats, less reliance on margarine, and the addition of liquid unsaturated vegetable oils.

Salt. Among the substances either found in foods or added to them that can affect your health is salt (sodium chloride). Most of us were brought up to eat and desire too much salt in our diets. From an early age, you probably enjoyed many commercially prepared and packaged foods, which contain great amounts of salt. I am often amazed at how people will sometimes grab the saltshaker before they have even tasted their food. Junk foods, such as potato chips, crackers, and pretzels, as well as prepared and smoked meats, have enormous quantities of salt and other sodium-containing substances.

High blood pressure (hypertension) is one of the major medical problems that affects people in Western countries. As you grow older, your blood pressure may increase. It appears that one of the factors determining the level of your blood pressure is the amount of salt that you consume. Even if you do not have high blood pressure, you should make a major effort to decrease the amount of salt in your diet. It will probably have a beneficial effect on your blood vessels as well as your heart. Learn to read labels on food products and avoid those products that show a high salt and sodium content. Develop the taste for other spices in your cooking. Stay away from junk foods, which not only have little food value and contain excessive amounts of salt, but are almost always fattening.

Alcohol. Although considered a beverage, *alcohol* is in fact a high-calorie food. Your attitude toward alcohol depends on how you look at the world. If you have strong feelings against alcohol, the thought of consuming any at all may be abhorrent to you. If, on the other hand, you have always enjoyed a drink or two, stopping altogether may be completely unacceptable.

There is abundant information about the deleterious effects of alcohol on the body. Excessive amounts can cause serious illnesses affecting the brain, nerves, liver, and heart. Almost everyone has known someone who "did himself in" with drink. Unless you are drinking fairly large amounts of alcohol, however, there is little danger that this will happen to you. But if you are drinking more than you used to, you should ask your physician for advice.

Alcohol is an "empty" source of calories: It is fattening and has no other nutritional value other than the calories themselves. If you tend to be unhappy or depressed, alcohol can exaggerate your feelings of despondency, despair, and isolation. In fact, all too often a depressed older person tries to use alcohol to feel better and instead begins to drink excessively. Mixing alcoholic drinks with some of the medications that you may require can be dangerous or even lethal.

On the bright side, some evidence shows that small amounts of alcohol, perhaps one drink a day, may have a beneficial effect on your heart. Certainly, you may find that your appetite will improve, and your desire to eat in company and share your meal will be enhanced by a small alcoholic drink before eating. When used judiciously and carefully, alcohol can enhance your well-being. If you drink, do so with the same caution that you would use with any other drug. Know its benefits and avoid its side effects.

Fiber. During the past several years, there has been a growing awareness of the importance of *dietary fiber* (roughage). The portion of vegetables and whole grains that is not digested is what is usually referred to as fiber. Because these substances are not absorbed by the body, it was assumed that they did not play an important role in our health. In fact, for many years the commercial preparation of foods placed a great deal of emphasis on removing fiber from foods. Therefore, we have been used to eating low-fiber diets.

It is now becoming clear that a lack of fiber in your diet may have a deleterious effect on your health. The most common symptom that results from a low-fiber diet is chronic *constipation*. Many older people are addicted to various forms of laxatives because of a lifetime of eating a low-fiber diet. A low-fiber diet has been implicated in diverticular disease of the colon, malignancies of the intestine, gallstones, and diabetes mellitus. Whether or not it will cure all your ills, you should gradually increase the amount of fiber in your diet. It should be done slowly, because if you have been used to a low-fiber diet for many years, a sudden increase in the amount may cause irritating and loose bowel movements.

The best sources of dietary fiber are *whole-grain cereals* that have not been overprocessed and *bran*. Commercial cereals that contain an adequate amount of fiber are still difficult to find, but some products are available. Read the labels carefully and look for the amounts of whole-grain cereal in the product.

Bran, a very important and readily available source of fiber, can be sprinkled on cooked and dry cereals and added to muffins and other homemade baked goods. Use it instead of bread crumbs in meatloaf and hamburgers, and cover poultry with it before broiling. Replace white bread with *whole-wheat bread*. This is an easy way to increase the amount of fiber in your diet. Raw vegetables and fruits are a welcome addition to any diet that has been low in fiber. If you have required laxatives for years, you will find that with a properly balanced high-fiber diet you can reduce or eliminate them. The other beneficial effects may be difficult to prove, but in all likelihood your general state of health will improve if you increase your fiber intake.

There is usually little interference between food and medications. Some drugs, such as tetracycline or erythromycin, may impair your appetite or make you nauseated. Others, such as quinidine, may give you diarrhea. This may impede your normal eating habits. It is important to ask your physician whether or not your medications should be taken before, during, or after meals. Some medications work best on an empty stomach, whereas others may cause nausea if taken without food.

Many medications can interfere with the metabolism or absorption of important nutrients. Diuretics may increase your need for potassium, which is found in citrus fruits and bananas. Large and frequent amounts of mineral oil may interfere with your absorption of vitamins A, D, E, and K. Some antibiotics may disrupt the normal workings of your bowel. Antacids can interfere with the absorption of phosphorus and may interfere with normal calcium metabolism and lead to weakened bones.

It is not always certain what the effect of different drugs will be on your diet and metabolism. It is important to clarify with your physician what precautions should be exercised when you are taking medications. He may recommend certain dietary supplements in order to ensure adequate nutrition.

The choice and variety of foods seems unlimited. By using simple principles, you can prepare attractive, nutritious, balanced, and tasteful meals. As a guide, *each day* you should try to have the following:

1 serving during *each* meal of a whole-grain cereal or whole-grain bread or macaroni product.

2 glasses of milk or its equivalent, such as yogurt, milk shake, custard, ice cream, cheese, or other milk product.

2 servings of high-quality protein, such as beef, fish, poultry, eggs, or vegetable protein from nuts and legumes, such as peas and beans. Try to avoid fatty meats such as pork, although occasionally they can be eaten.

2 servings of fruit, including one with a high content of vitamin C.

2 servings of vegetables, preferably fresh, which should include salad greens. Vegetables should be slightly boiled,

steamed, or baked. Avoid overboiling because the vitamins are lost in the water.

8 glasses of liquids, including water, juices, soups, and watery fruits.

Drink tea and coffee in moderation.

One serving of bread is one slice, and one serving of cereal is about one-third to one-half a cup. A serving of fruit usually means one whole small fruit or one-half cup, depending on its form. A vegetable serving is one-half cup. A serving of meat or other protein is three ounces.

It is best to divide your meals over five or six small portions per day. This can include a few in-between snacks of low-salt crackers, cheese, and fruits. Avoid all types of pre-prepared foods whenever possible, and stay away from junk foods.

With this as a guide, you should be able to have a well-balanced and attractive diet.

VITAMIN SUPPLEMENTS

Vitamins are found in many varieties of foods and in small quantities are essential for health. Absence of any one vitamin can lead to an illness because these substances are necessary for important steps of metabolism. The diseases caused by vitamin lack are called *deficiency states. Scurvy* due to an extreme lack of vitamin C and rickets caused by vitamin D deficiency are well-known examples of this type of disorder. However, extra amounts of vitamins do not necessarily improve health or prevent disease. In fact, some vitamins in excess can be toxic.

The manufacturing and marketing of supplemental vitamins and minerals is a major industry. Magazine articles, television commercials, and books often extol the merits of one type of vitamin supplement or another. Some people, including some health care personnel, recommend vitamin supplements in massive doses, known as *megavitamins.* Some people claim that one vitamin or another can prevent cancer, restore health, regrow hair, reawaken sexual drive, or improve many of the processes that seem to wane as you grow older. However, no vitamin has ever been shown conclusively to increase life or health if given in greater than normal amounts.

Most vitamins have been studied in great detail over many years, so we have a good idea as to how they work and the amounts necessary for normal human function. Some new important information is coming out of investigations on older persons as to requirements and deficiencies. Many of the previous studies were done on younger people. So far, however, there has not been a striking difference between your vitamin and mineral needs as you grow older than when you were younger. Some evidence suggests that in some older people, especially those with severe illnesses or those requiring numerous medications, the absorption of some vitamins may be impaired. In these cases greater amounts than usual may be required to maintain an adequate level in your body.

Therefore, in general, if your health is good and you are not taking numerous medications, your absorption of the vitamins normally found in a well-balanced diet should be sufficient to maintain your health. You may want to take a supplemental multiple vitamin either because you "believe" or your doctor "believes" that this will make up for any deficiencies in your diet. If you would like to take a vitamin supplement, ask your physician to prescribe one that takes into account your own needs. Many commercial products have little in the way of nutritional value and are considerably overpriced.

I met one elderly woman who was opening a parcel from her pharmacy. She was about to pay the delivery boy a fairly large sum of money when I asked her if I could look at the bottle. It contained a liquid vitamin "tonic" supposedly designed for the older person. The vitamin content was in fact less than the standard multiple vitamin tablet that could be purchased at approximately one-tenth the price. It was contained in what smelled like sherry. I told the lady that she could receive a prescription for a month's supply of multiple vitamins and buy two bottles of quality sherry for the amount she was spending for a two-week supply of this "tonic." The appetite-stimulant effect of the "tonic" was no doubt because of the sherry. Her well-being and good appetite continued when she switched to the tablets and took a small glass of good sherry before her main meal. She donated the difference in cost to charity.

VITAMIN C

There has been at least as much written about vitamin C as any other vitamin known to man. Great quantities are consumed daily by millions of people whose hope is that it will increase their defenses against infection and somehow improve their skin and the function of their heart and blood vessels, among other things.

Vitamin C is found abundantly in fresh fruit, especially citrus fruits. It is found generously in melons, strawberries, and fresh vegetables, such as green peppers, cabbage, tomatoes, and spinach. Other vegetables that contain considerable quantities of vitamin C include broccoli, brussels sprouts, cauliflower, peas, and potatoes. When vegetables are overboiled, however, this water-soluable vitamin may leak into the liquid, thereby leaving relatively little in the vegetable. This can be overcome by steaming your vegetables rather than boiling them, or by using a small amount of water, which you can then save and add to soup.

Many studies have attempted to show that adding vitamin C to your diet will increase your level of general health and longevity. A number have tried to prove that large doses of vitamin C improve your resistance to respiratory disease and decrease the effect and duration of some infectious illnesses, particularly colds. Other than some evidence suggesting that it may promote an increased resistance to colds, there has been little firm support that vitamin C will improve your general level of health or increase your lifespan. The doses recommended for this purpose are usually ten to forty times the amounts that are known to be necessary for normal metabolism, which is about 50 milligrams per day. Although excess amounts of vitamin C have few side effects, some people experience burning when passing urine.

Unless you have a specific ailment that interferes with your normal absorption of vitamin C, or you cannot eat enough fruits and vegetables, there is no need to take the vitamin as a nutritional supplement. There is little evidence to suggest that large doses (500 mg. to 2 grams) taken daily are in any way beneficial to your heart, blood vessels, lungs, or body in general. Taking such large doses of vitamin C at the beginning of or during a cold may have some benefit in decreasing the symptoms and its duration, however.

If you are plagued by frequent respiratory infections, it would be prudent to see your physician first about other factors that might be making you susceptible. Certainly it is more important for you to stop smoking than to take a vitamin C pill in order to improve your lung function and prevent infection.

Research is being conducted to determine whether supplemental vitamin C and vitamin E will decrease the incidence of gastrointestinal cancer. It has been determined that, in countries where little C and E are consumed, the incidence of gastrointestinal cancer is higher. In Western countries, large quantities of nitrates (nitrosamines) are eaten; they are used abundantly in preserved and smoked meats, and some researchers believe that they may be carcinogenic (cancer-forming) if eaten for many years. It is possible, however, that large doses of vitamin C and vitamin E can inhibit the nitrates from becoming carcinogenic. Until the research is completed, it is probably more reasonable to decrease the amount of nitrates in your diet rather than take excessively large amounts of these two vitamins. A well-balanced diet with ample vegetables, fruits, and juices is more likely to assure your good health than taking supplemental vitamin C.

VITAMIN E

Vitamin E is one of the vitamins most commonly taken by the elderly, and its production, promotion, and sale is a multimillion-dollar industry.

Vitamin E is found most commonly in fats, especially in vegetable fats. Cereals and other grain products, dairy products, fish, meat, eggs, and green, leafy vegetables also contain considerable amounts. The body absorbs it well, and because it is a fat-soluble vitamin, it is efficiently stored in the body. Vitamin E deficiency in experimental animals has been found when E is purposely removed from their diets. It is, however, very difficult to detect true vitamin E deficiency in human beings. Proponents of the beneficial affects of vitamin E claim that when taken in large amounts, it can prevent many human diseases. Although numerous reports over the years have claimed positive effects, few seem to be conclusive in their assessment of benefit to humans.

There are certain childhood diseases for which vitamin E seems beneficial, and adults who suffer from cirrhosis of the liver, certain types of pancreatic disease, and illnesses leading to malabsorption of fats may derive some benefit. But only because they cannot adequately absorb this substance should they take it in large quantities.

Many claims have been made that vitamin E has a beneficial affect on circulation. Some studies done on the heart and blood vessels show that people who suffer from pain in their legs because of an inadequate blood supply (intermittent claudication) may benefit from vitamin E. However, the response to vitamin E therapy is not universal. If you suffer from intermittent claudication and have not benefited from other medications or from surgery, you may experience some relief of symptoms with vitamin E in a dosage of 400 to 800 International Units (IU) daily.

Vitamin E has been claimed to improve sexual function, muscle strength, and athletic ability, as well as decrease the symptoms of angina pectoris and coronary heart disease and retard the aging process. However, there is no conclusive evidence of this. Nevertheless, you may still be convinced that vitamin E works. Many popular books recommend its use for all kinds of problems associated with aging, so it may be difficult to convince you that vitamin E is unnecessary.

One eminent professor of cardiology tells the story about his patients, many of whom, by the time they came to see him for consultation, were already taking large doses of vitamin E. In the early days of his practice he would tell them that the vitamin was not necessary. When some of these patients developed heart attacks, they would say to him, "See, that's what happens when you stop taking vitamin E."

On one occasion he saw a patient who had previously been raving about the beneficial effects of vitamin E on his angina pectoris. The man subsequently suffered a heart attack. The professor remarked when he saw him, "Well, I guess the vitamin E didn't really help." The patient looked at him discouragingly and said, "To tell you the truth, Doc, I probably wasn't taking enough."

A recent article in a major medical journal described the results of a study done under the auspices of the U.S. Public Health Service over a six-month period. It failed to show any positive effect of vitamin E on the symptoms of angina pectoris or coronary artery disease. Other than those who suffer from a problem with the absorption of food or perhaps who have symptoms related to an impaired blood supply to the legs, there does not appear to be a need to take vitamin E supplements.

It is often claimed that vitamin E has never been shown to cause serious side effects. This is not so. Some physicians claim that an excess can increase your tendency to form blood clots in your legs *(thrombophlebitis)*. Other side effects may be fatigue, muscle weakness, skin rash, and breast tenderness. Therefore, you cannot justify taking vitamin E by saying, "At least it can't do any harm." All unnecessary medications can do harm, physically, financially, or by lulling you into a false sense of security that may keep you from taking other important steps in your health care.

Taking vitamin E supplements is an expensive way to try to promote your health and longevity. Further research may demonstrate some positive effects of this vitamin, but until then vitamin E is not necessary as a dietary supplement.

HEALTH FOODS

Most communities have at least one health-food store. In addition to food products, many of these shops also sell vitamins and other food supplements. Many people are attracted to them because they think the products are of higher quality or "purer" than those found in local stores or supermarkets.

Some aspects of health-food stores may be helpful if you are trying to maintain a balanced and nutritious diet. Unlike most supermarkets, *small quantities* of food can usually be purchased, and they carry items that do not contain as many additives and preservatives as commercially prepared products. Of course, not all food additives are harmful; however, some found in many commercial foods are unnecessary.

Decreasing the amount of salt and sugar in your diet is desirable as you grow older. When you read the labels of many commercially prepared cereals and breads, you will find that they often contain excessive amounts of both. Health-food stores usually have cereals and breads that contain little or no salt and sugar. But be aware that "sea salt" and honey have many of the same deleterious effects as table salt and refined sugar. Do not assume that you can eat unlimited quantities of these products just because they are sold in health-food stores.

However, there should be a place in your diet for whole-grain cereals and breads, nuts, and dried fruits, such as dates, figs, prunes, and apricots. These can usually be purchased without unnecessary additives. You can also find cheese, yogurt, and other dairy products without salt, sugar, and preservatives. These may be more appropriate for your diet than similar products sold elsewhere.

One product that I often recommend is the *granola-type* cereal. You can also buy the ingredients separately and mix them yourself. They are a useful source of the *B complex* vitamins and natural fiber and do not contain sugar, salt, or preservatives. They make a tasty and nutritious breakfast cereal and can also be used in cooking and baking. Peanut butter without sugar, salt, corn syrup and hydrogenated oils is also a good source of vegetable protein.

The vitamins and various food supplements sold in health-food stores are usually not necessary to ensure your good health and nutrition. Sometimes they may even be harmful, particularly when taken in large quantities. Their quality control may be below standard, and they may contain substances that you cannot tolerate.

Judiciously buying small quantities of good quality cereals, nuts, breads, dried fruits, juices, and dairy products can be economical, but some products are more expensive in these stores. Examine the products and the labels carefully and choose those items that are economical and useful to ensure a well-balanced diet.

SEXUAL FEELINGS

A great deal has been written and spoken about sexuality in the aging person. This is not surprising in a society that has become more open about discussing its sexual feelings. In some ways you may both benefit and suffer from the new freedom of sexual expression. Many older people have ideas about their sexuality that are quite different from those of the younger generation. You were brought up at a time when sex was not discussed openly, and there was less physical freedom. With this background you may not be able to adapt easily to new sexual attitudes. Many people have never had the opportunity to express their sexual feelings. You might feel somewhat inhibited about discussing them, even though you might welcome the chance to act on your sexual inclinations.

Many myths about the sexual needs and abilities of the elderly are held by most younger people and by many health care professionals, including physicians and nurses. Because of these traditional beliefs, you may find it difficult to express your sexual needs or feel comfortable with them. One common myth is that sexual desire and attraction decrease with age. But youth does not have a monopoly on sex. Although books, television, and movies almost never depict an older person expressing passion or love, this is just a reflection of the myth.

Another myth is that as you grow older your body does not need or respond to sexual desire. It is assumed somehow that your sexual organs stop functioning and you forget about sex after you reach some mysterious age. I have observed that most people continue to have the same pattern of sexual expression and desire that they had during their younger years. Those who were reserved and not particularly sexually active will probably find it quite easy to assume a more sedate sexual life. You may not even regret the lack of a sexual outlet. This is especially so If during your sexually active years you merely tolerated sex and had little enjoyment of it.

People who were sexually active during youth and derived enjoyment from it will probably continue to do so. If you have a suitable partner, you will probably continue to have an active sex life into your old age. You may find that some of your physical needs and abilities have changed, but you will learn to modify your sexual activities to fit your abilities. In some ways sexual activity is like riding a bicycle. Once you learn, you never forget how. The problem is that you may not always have a bicycle handy, or the models change and the new ones are not quite the same. However, if you persist, you will probably be able to accommodate to the changing times and continue to derive pleasure from sex.

Younger people often feel that sex is not proper or moral for the older person. One often hears an older gentleman referred to as a "dirty old man" if he verbally or physically expresses appreciation of or attraction to a younger female. This is unfortunate, since such activities by a younger man would no doubt be praised. These responses often seem to occur in hospitals and other institutional settings.

It is most important for you to be able to express comfortably your affection and sexuality. Your family, physician, and other health professionals should be cautioned about pushing you if you are not ready to deal with these feelings, however. Some of us in the medical profession may overact in our zeal to allow the older individual to reveal sexual needs. One elderly widow was appalled when her physician thoughtfully and tactfully asked if she was having sexual feelings when she complained of persistent discomfort around her vagina. The woman was so insulted that her physician would think such a thing so many years after her beloved husband's death that she refused to see that doctor ever again. Although this was an exaggerated response, it could be understood in terms of this woman's lifelong view of sex in relationship to her late husband.

Your sexual requirements and ability to fulfill them depend on many factors. Those with a sexual partner, either through marriage or another arrangement, will probably have an easier time expressing particular sexual needs than those who are alone. However, even young couples can have problems that inhibit each member from being able to fulfill individual needs. Nevertheless, if you have had a long relationship and have weathered the storms of life together, you should be able to explore your mutual sexual needs.

Many people are reticent about discussing their sexual feelings with each other. This is especially so if they have not been used to doing it before. Most people certainly cannot discuss their inclinations with their children because most children continue to be amazed that their older parents "indulge" in sex. Some physicians hold the same ideas and may not be sympathetic or approachable. Many physicians, however, will respond to your concerns or will refer you to a qualified counselor who can help you work out your sexual problems.

For those without a permanent sexual partner, fulfilling your sexual needs is more difficult. The "double standard" exists even for the elderly. A single man usually can find a suitable sexual partner at any age. So long as you are a healthy and sexually active man, there is a strong likelihood that a female partner will be available. Women, on the other hand, have more difficulty finding appropriate partners as they grow older, especially since they outnumber men. And older women usually will not take the initiative as readily in finding a partner. Also, single older men can accept sexual encounters more easily outside the framework of marriage. As a hangover from previously held standards, older women will often avoid sexual involvements outside of marriage. With changing attitudes, however, women may no longer have to wait until a man finds them. There are more and more opportunities at social clubs and other senior-citizen centers for you to discover partners suitable for your emotional and sexual needs.

Many general myths about sexuality become even more exaggerated as you grow older. You may believe them, your children may accept them, and many physicians assume them. But you may be able to overcome the power and influence of these myths if you receive proper advice about them. Many people assume that sexual desire is lost after menopause. Although menopause is referred to as the "change of life," this does not necessarily mean that your sexual needs and desires will change too. Many aspects of menopause, both physical and emotional, may lead to some changes in your sexual inclinations. You may feel less attractive to your partner because you associate menopause with "growing old." Your partner may also react negatively if he is not aware of the normal changes that occur during this period of life. You may begin to feel worthless, if you connect your value as a woman with your ability to have children. You may fear that your partner will look elsewhere to younger, fertile women for sexual fulfillment.

Many women experience several menopausal symptoms, including depression, flushes, perspiring, and a general loss of motivation. These symptoms can aggravate your emotional feelings and cause you to turn away from sex. This, in turn, reinforces your partner's belief that after menopause sexual needs and abilities decrease in women. You may even try the opposite approach and become more sexually active in an attempt to overcome your fears. This, too, can lead to uncomfortable sexual interactions if your partner is not aware of why this is happening.

Menopause does not change your ability to have and enjoy sex. The fact that you are no longer fertile does not interfere with your ability to respond sexually or to delight in the same physical rewards of intimacy that you enjoyed previously. If your menopausal symptoms are pronounced, many physicians will prescribe small doses of female hormones, which may improve both your physical and emotional feelings.

If you have had a hysterectomy, you may also feel that your ability for sexual fulfillment will be curtailed. Your reproductive organs have nothing to do with the physical or emotional aspects of sexual enjoyment. After they are removed, you should be able to return to normal sexual activity. If the surgery has somehow affected your vagina, you should ask your physician how it can be treated. Some women may develop a painful thinning of the lining of the vagina many years after menopause or after a total hysterectomy. You may require some assistance in proper vaginal lubrication. Rather than experiencing pain during intercourse, consult your physician about how to achieve proper lubrication. Some women benefit from small amounts of locally applied female hormone cream (estrogen) or lubricant jelly.

Although men appear to be less obviously affected by aging, they also suffer sexual problems. You may not have difficulty finding suitable partners either because you are already married or because, despite being single, many women are available. However, you may discover that your capability for sexual activity has deteriorated. This can be very frightening and frustrating and may lead to a diminished sexual interest.

Many older men who have had surgery on their prostate gland think that they will no longer be able to be active sexually. Your physician should dispel this misconception, however. It is unusual for prostate surgery to effect your physical ability to have sexual fulfillment permanently. However, this type of surgery as well as many other physical and emotional stresses can sometimes impair your sexual capacity.

The problem of *impotence* in elderly men is common. It may be difficult to tell your partner, and you may avoid sex altogether rather than admit your inability to perform. You may not be able to express your problem to your doctor either, especially if you feel he is unsympathetic. Some people try over-the-counter medicines to improve sexuality, but most are ineffective and only postpone finding a proper solution.

Although a few well-known medical conditions can interfere with your ability to have an erection and achieve sexual fulfillment, for the most part these are not the common causes of impotence. You must explain your condition to your physician. Your health should be evaluated so that illnesses and medications that might interfere with sexual activity and sexual feelings can be controlled. An illness, such as diabetes, and certain drugs, such as those for high blood pressure, as well as tranquilizers and sedatives, may interfere with sexual function.

For many men impotence is a psychological problem. You may have developed a fear of failing, perhaps because you have a younger sexual partner whom you suspect may not be faithful to you. You might be experiencing marital problems and have unconsciously responded with impotence. You may have fears about your financial situation, your work, or any number of other things. Sometimes impotence occurs after a major physical illness. If you had a heart attack, you may be terrified of having sex again, fearing that such excitement could bring on another heart attack. This may show itself as impotence, and you should consult your physician. If, for example, physical excitement leads to an attack of angina pectoris, your physician may recommend that you take a nitroglycerin tablet fifteen to twenty minutes before sexual activity. Such problems should be openly discussed with your physician and your partner.

Some physicians prescribe *testosterone* (male hormone) tablets or injections for impotence. In some men impotence may be the result of a decrease or lack of this hormone. Until now the degree of success with hormone treatment has not been as great as would be expected. Those who do improve with this medication should take it for only a short time, for it can have adverse effects on your prostate gland.

Some urologists (specialist of kidneys, bladder, prostate) have taken on the additional role of sexual counselor. Psychiatrists can also be helpful. Most impotent men will respond to proper counseling. Your family physician may be the most appropriate person for this kind of help because he probably knows you better than others, and he may also understand your marital situation. If he is not sympathetic to your needs, find someone who is. Most men suffering from impotence respond to treatment and return to a reasonably active and satisfying sexual life.

Although your basic attitudes and inclinations toward sexuality will not change as you grow older, some alterations in ability may occur. You may notice that your sex drive has decreased, or arousal and intercourse might become less important than physical closeness, hugging, and touching. You probably will need physical intimacy as much as when you were younger, and you should allow yourself to express this need. If you and your partner find that you have different needs, you must learn to discuss it together. Sometimes sexual counseling will help in this case too.

One elderly woman who was about to be remarried saw one of my colleagues for advice. After discussing the good points of her future partner, she ventured some questions as to their sexual possibilities. The physician recommended the use of a vaginal lubricant before intercourse and encouraged her to relax and learn to express her feelings positively. At the end of the visit, she eagerly commented, "As I remember it, I used to like it and I think I was pretty good at it." In fact, their marriage has succeeded, both emotionally and physically.

For some people the only obstacle to satisfying sexual expression is not having a suitable partner, and the isolation and loss of physical contact may be very disturbing. Many older people have a very negative attitude toward *masturbation.* You were brought up at a time when masturbation was looked upon as sinful or perverted. It may be virtually impossible for you to start masturbating now if you did not when you were younger. Unfortunately, some physicians share the same negative attitude, but there are increasing numbers of sex counselors with more positive attitudes who can be consulted.

Masturbation can be a useful and satisfying way of achieving some degree of sexual satisfaction. You may have to learn how if you were not used to doing it before. Most people at some point in their lives have masturbated, and it is an acknowledged *normal* process in sexual development. But you may have had such negative feelings toward it for religious or moral reasons that you may have shunned it completely. If you are not opposed to trying it again, you should know that as you grow older it may take longer for you to reach a level of self-arousal. You must be gentle with yourself, and if excess friction is required to achieve satisfaction, a small amount of lubricant jelly may be helpful, in both women and men.

There are many people who have a partner, but for some reason, full sexual relations may not be possible. Perhaps health problems interfere. If you feel comfortable with each other, and sometimes with the help of a counselor, you may discover that massage, caressing, and masturbation of each other can be a satisfactory way of achieving mutual sexual satisfaction. Do not be afraid to express your needs and experiment. You will probably be relieved to find that you can achieve sexual fulfillment without feeling guilty.

For some, the prime physical contacts and ways of expressing sexual feelings are through friends and family. Hugs, kisses, and touching become necessary substitutes for more direct sexual activity. Talking is very important. You should express your feelings and not be afraid to admire the sexual development of your children and grandchildren. Touching and holding them, experiencing their growth and development, is a marvelous addition to your own sexual feelings. Enjoy whatever you can. Warmth and emotional satisfaction enhance the fulfillment of sexual needs.

LIVING ARRANGEMENTS

There is no doubt that most of us would like to live out our later years in our own homes with their many memories. We are all aware that nursing homes and hospitals are necessary for the poor, sick, and lonely, but we assume, as we often do about illness and death, that these are things that happen to others and not to ourselves.

Most of us have had to make numerous decisions in our lives about where we are going to live. Many people have lived in several places, either in one city or town or in many geographic locations. You may be near members of your family, or you may be far removed from them. At some point, you may have to examine whether your living arrangement is the best one for you now and in the future.

Some changes in living arrangements may be precipitated by illnesses, whereas others are made by changes in social, financial, and family needs. The alterations that follow an illness are more difficult to deal with because usually there has been no planning or forethought about them. Other changes may have been considered for many years before the move finally occurs.

Usually, you move because you want to, rather than because you have no alternative.

If you are having difficulty maintaining yourself in your own home, you and your children may raise the possibility of moving into a nursing home, retirement community, or even a chronic hospital (for long-term care). The latter becomes an issue only if you have become too ill or dependent to look after your most basic needs. The decision to move into a retirement community or nursing home must be based on many factors. You may resist the thought of relocating your lives and giving up the comfort, privacy, familiarity, and individuality of your own home, which cannot be supplied even by the best institution.

On the other hand, your home may have become a prison if you feel isolated and are physically or emotionally impaired. Perhaps some of your friends have died or left your neighborhood, and perhaps your family is scattered in distant places. The chores of shopping and housework can become overwhelming if your physical capabilities begin to fail. Your fear of illness or accident may become so great that you might not risk going outdoors. A sudden illness for which no one can be contacted may be so frightening a prospect that you may begin to fear being alone.

Ideally, with close family and friends nearby, you may be able to stay in your home or with a family member. In many cities and towns, community services can assist you at home. Meals on Wheels and visiting nurses, homemakers, and physicians may be enough to allow you to keep your home. Senior-citizen centers can assist you in remaining social and active and also assist your family, who may be looking after you. With this type of care, you will probably be happier at home.

If you feel imprisoned at home, however, moving into a retirement community or nursing home may be a welcome solution to your problem. The institution may satisfy not only your physical needs, but it also may allow a creative outlet.

In most communities there are more nursing homes than any other type of facility for the older person who can no longer live at home. Some nursing homes divide the type of care required for their residents between those who are more independent and those who are more needy. However, in many instances all the residents are in fairly close quarters, and this has disadvantages, of course.

If you are physically well and active, a retirement home or community may be more suitable. You may have to move from your old neighborhood or town, so the difficulty in maintaining contacts with friends and family has to be weighed against the benefits. Many older people and especially older couples are choosing to move to retirement communities in warmer climates. Here, too, you might be leaving family and friends, although these communities usually foster a strong neighborhood spirit. During times of crises it may be difficult to arrange for assistance and the comfort that a nearby family gives. Children often become disturbed by the thought that should an illness occur, they will not be able to help their parents. If you choose this type of living arrangement, try it out first if possible without making a firm commitment. Explore the facilities for both recreation and work. Speak to as many residents as you can, and make sure that the medical care is of high quality. When you move, ask your physician to forward your medical records to your new physician. Ask your doctor to keep a copy of your file in his office. If you return for a visit, you may still want or need his medical advice as well.

If you move into a nursing home in your vicinity, you or your children should explore the residence as thoroughly as possible. The type and quality of nursing homes vary according to regional, financial, social, and political factors. Unfortunately, some homes are badly supervised and poorly run. Others maintain an exceptionally high quality of care. Municipal homes vary in quality depending on the locale, but they may have more stringent regulations than commercial institutions. Many philanthropic organizations and religious groups support and organize homes for the aged. In my experience, they provide a consistently higher level of care than commercial nursing homes. Because they are sponsored by nonprofit organizations, their degree of commitment and responsibility is frequently greater than nonaffiliated nursing homes.

If you require a great deal of nursing and medical care, you may have to move to a hospital supplying long-term care. There are many types, depending on where you live. They vary in quality but usually give adequate care as well as provide some outlet for psychological and emotional needs.

Once you decide to move into a nursing or retirement home, find the best and most suitable one for you. You may have to rely on your family or health care professionals to assist you in making a decision. Depending on where you live, there may be a great deal of choice or little choice at all in finding a suitable home. If many residences are available, inspect them yourself or with a member of your family. Do not be afraid to speak to residents and their families, and ask the medical and nursing supervisors about the care that is given and the attitude of the staff.

It is important to determine the type of medical care you will receive. It is preferable to have a physician whose commitment to the home is permanent and stable, rather than having a "rotating" physician. You should be assured of the availability of your own physician too. An inspection of the kitchen is important, and ask if you could eat with the residents if possible. Social and recreational facilities are crucial. Ask the residents what programs are available and how often and how well they are arranged.

Your family should not be afraid to ask about the care that you will be given and what kind of access they will have to members of the social service and nursing and medical staff. It is important that at the time of admission, you and your family feel comfortable that the decision is the best one for all concerned. This cannot always be achieved, however. Your children may feel guilty and you may feel resentment. You could seek professional assistance to help ease you and your children through this difficult transition period.

Although many people feel that by entering a nursing or retirement home, they are on their last journey in life, the opposite is often the case. In well-run, creative facilities, your life may become more active and interesting than when you were living at home alone. Many good residences provide activities that may rekindle interests that were dormant for many years. I have met many older people who embarked on new paths of expression and creation after they had moved into such residences. You can make of it what you would like. You may have to work hard and commit yourself in the beginning, but you can adjust and continue to lead an interesting and satisfying life.

CHAPTER 5

Commonly Used Medications

Remembering the names of the various drugs that you may be taking can be very confusing. It is difficult enough to try to understand why each medication was prescribed. What complicates even the most heroic attempt to keep track of medications is the fact that many of them appear to be similar, and they not only have strange names, but they may be called by various terms.

Every medication has an official, or *generic,* name. This is the general term used by all the companies that produce it, and usually the term is international. In addition, generic drugs have many *trade*® *names,* according to which firm markets them. The trade names may also vary from country to country. Therefore, a drug with a generic name may have five or six different trade names.

GENERIC VERSUS TRADE NAMES

The problem of multiple names can cause severe complications when similar drugs are taken at the same time, particularly if they have been prescribed in different dosages. For instance, a commonly used tranquilizer is called *diazepam* by its generic name, but it is also sold as Valium®, Vivol®, D-Tran®, E-Pam®, Erital®, Meval®, Novodipam®, Paxel®, Neo-Calme®, Stress-Pam®, Apaurin®, Lembrol®, Setonil®, and many others. To confuse the issue even more, there are many derivatives of diazepam with different generic names and trade names, but they all do the same thing. For instance, the generic tranquilizer *oxazepam* is sold under the names Serax®, Adumbran®, Limbial®, and Seresta®, among others, but it is similar to diazepam.

Whenever your physician prescribes a medication, always ask its generic name and the family of drugs to which it belongs. For instance, if you are given a medication in the family of *steroids,* you should be made aware that this is a drug that mimics the action of *cortisone.* There are many members of the steroid class of drugs and, if you are receiving one, it is of utmost importance that you know because special precautions must be taken (see page 362).

At the pharmacy make sure that the generic term is written on the label in addition to the trade name. Also, ask your pharmacist if you are receiving any other medication in the same family to ensure that two similar drugs have not been inadvertently prescribed. For this reason it is very important always to use the same pharmacist. Since it would be impossible to discuss every medication used to treat the many illnesses that can affect you, the following compendium will note the most common types and families of drugs and their *generic* names. No mention will be made of trade names, as they vary so widely.

A COMPENDIUM OF DRUGS

Analgesic medications are used to dispel pain, but some have other effects as well. For example, *aspirin,* a good painkiller, lowers an elevated temperature and has an effective antiinflammatory action. Some of its success in relieving the pain of arthritic conditions is because of its antiinflammatory effect, in addition to its analgesic action. Aspirin (salicylate) is sold in many forms, by prescription and over the counter. It is useful for many forms of pain affecting the muscles and bones. The most common side effect is an upset of the intestinal tract, and it may cause irritation and bleeding in the stomach. Some people experience a ringing in their ears when excess amounts are taken. Aspirin has many other uses in addition to analgesia: It decreases the stickiness of the blood (tendency for blood to clot) and is presently being used in the treatment and prevention of strokes.

Other analgesics are often prescribed for those who cannot tolerate aspirin but require treatment for pain. The milder medications that can be bought over the counter include acetaminophen, which may also help lower fever, as does aspirin. Although it was once thought to be relatively harmless, when taken in excess, it can have deleterious effects on the liver. Propoxyphene, widely sold as a mild analgesic, can cause dizziness or fainting and should not be taken with alcohol. Codeine in most countries must be obtained through a doctor's prescription. However, in some places small doses can be bought over the counter. Codeine can cause a number of problems in the elderly, including constipation and mental confusion.

The more potent analgesics, called opiates include morphine and meperidine. These substances are used only for short periods, such as for an injury or after surgery. They also play an important role in the treatment of malignant disease. In many instances these drugs are addicting and will cause a clouding of consciousness and lead to drowsiness or mental confusion. They must always be used under medical supervision.

The pain of arthritis and rheumatism, although sometimes relieved by analgesics, is usually more effectively treated with antiinflammatory drugs. The most important and best-known, of course, is aspirin. For inflammatory disorders, however, aspirin may be needed in much larger quantities than when used to treat other types of pain. There are a number of new medications called *nonsteroidal antiinflammatory* drugs, used for the treatment of arthritis. Some of the older drugs in this group, such as *phenylbutazone* and *indomethacin,* are very effective, but they may cause a severe gastrointestinal upset similar to aspirin. The exact place of the newer antiinflammatory drugs is now being established. Today, it is common for patients to be prescribed one of the newer forms of these medications. For this reason it is especially important to check with your physician to see whether a similar drug is being used simultaneously for the same purpose.

Cortisone-like drugs (steroids), such as *prednisone* are also used for inflammatory diseases. These medications have many serious side effects, but their use may at times be necessary and even life-saving. Their administration must be carefully supervised by a physician.

For special kinds of arthritis, such as gout or pseudogout, other medications may be useful that are not effective for other arthritic conditions. *Colchicine* is often used during an acute attack of gout, either by mouth or by injection. It can cause diarrhea, but this improves as soon as the dosage is decreased. After an acute episode of gout is treated with colchicine or other antiinflammatory medication, further attacks may be prevented with *allopurinol,* which decreases the formation of uric acid. On rare occasions it can cause a severe skin rash, but this usually improves when the drug is stopped.

Medications to treat heart disease are commonly prescribed for older individuals. The main disorders of the heart are those of abnormal rhythms, poor oxygen supply, and failure of the heart to pump effectively. The drugs that regulate these disorders fall into various categories; some have multiple effects and are often used in combination with others.

The most commonly prescribed drug for the heart is *digoxin.* In most countries only one manufacturer markets digoxin because in the past there was a problem in the drug's consistency when it was produced by different companies. The generic name is digoxin, but its trade name is Lanoxin®. This drug has a number of effects on the heart. It improves the pumping strength and therefore is useful in treating heart failure. In addition, it affects the heart's rhythm and is often used to control certain types of abnormal and irregular heart rhythms. Sometimes both effects are needed simultaneously.

Digoxin can have serious side effects. The amount required in older people and those with kidney disorders is often less than in younger individuals. The first side effect of excessive dosage is nausea and impaired appetite, and occasionally mental confusion. In addition, some older men may experience a swelling of the breasts. However, the most serious complication is a toxic abnormality of the heart's rhythm different from those it is used to treat. Therefore, this drug must be used *only* under careful medical supervision. An extra dose should never be taken on your own.

Abnormal heart rhythms can cause many symptoms in the elderly. In addition to digoxin, *quinidine* is also effective for their control. Its side effects include nausea, vomiting, diarrhea, dizziness, and sometimes blood disorders, and many older people cannot tolerate it at all. *Procainamide,* used in the same fashion, can cause similar problems and must be taken even more frequently. It is often inconvenient for an older person because a nighttime dose is usually necessary for the drug to be effective. However, a long-acting preparation is now available, which may make it more useful, as the doses can be given less often.

A new product, *disopyramide,* is effective for heart-rhythm disorders. It has fewer side effects than quinidine, but it often causes an uncomfortable dryness in the mouth. In men, especially if they have prostate problems, it may cause the flow of urine to decrease or sometimes stop. However, this is reversible when the drug is discontinued.

A number of medications used for the treatment of angina pectoris work by increasing the efficiency of the heart and decreasing its need for oxygen. Some drugs also cause some of the coronary blood vessels to dilate and thereby carry more blood. *Nitroglycerin* was the first drug in the family of *nitrates* that was used for angina pectoris. It is placed under the tongue, where it dissolves, and usually it is taken every few hours or when symptoms of angina pectoris occur. Allowing a tablet of nitroglycerin to dissolve *before* physical activity rather than after will often prevent an attack of anginal pain.

Many *long-acting nitrates* can be taken either as tablets or dissolved under the tongue. The most common is *isosorbide dinitrate,* which has many trade names. Sometimes combinations of these medications may be employed, with the long-acting varieties being taken every few hours and nitroglycerin used when there is an exaggeration of discomfort. An *ointment of nitroglycerin* is also useful, especially at night if symptoms occur. All of the nitrates can cause a feeling of fullness or a pounding in the head. This usually improves with time or if the dose is decreased for a few days and then increased. Some people become dizzy, or their blood pressure may fall. It is unusual for a person not to be able to tolerate at least a small dose, however.

Propranolol, one of the many *beta-blockers,* serves many purposes. The beta-blockers interfere with the effect of adrenaline on the heart, preventing an unnecessary increase in the speed and effort of the heart. Aside from the effect on angina pectoris and hypertension, propranolol can prevent and control certain kinds of abnormal heart rhythms. It can be used alone or in conjunction with digoxin, quinidine, or disopyramide. Usually, it is taken from two to four times daily. It slows the pulse, and some people may develop an inordinately slow heart rate. In patients with asthma or chronic bronchitis, it may exaggerate wheezing. And in certain individuals, it may aggravate the symptoms of heart failure.

Medications used to treat *hypertension* (high blood pressure) often overlap with those used for various forms of heart disease. *Diuretics* ("water pills") are medications that cause the body to lose salt and water. In people who suffer from heart failure, there is an excessive accumulation of fluid because of impaired pumping of the heart. Diuretics allow the excess fluid to be passed through the kidneys and thereby decrease the shortness of breath, bloating, and swelling.

It may be necessary to use diuretics with other medications when high blood pressure is difficult to control. The most common diuretics, the *thiazides,* come in many forms, as individual medications and sometimes in combination with other drugs. They are slow acting and rarely create an urgency to urinate, as do the faster-acting diuretics, such as *furosemide.* The fast-acting diuretics are more potent than the thiazides for the treatment of heart failure but are not more effective in treating high blood pressure. The diuretics *spiranolactone* and *triamterene* are often combined with other diuretics to enhance their effect and prevent excessive loss of potassium, which is often a problem with the other types of medications. Sometimes *potassium* tablets or syrup may be given with thiazides or furosemide. Potassium should not be taken if you are receiving spiranolactone or triamterene.

These medications may cause an excessive loss of salt and water, which can lead to dizziness and fainting, or they may decrease the efficiency of the kidneys. In people who have a tendency to diabetes mellitus, diuretics may increase the level of sugar in the blood (see page 364). In certain individuals gout may occur. If you are taking diuretics, expect to have periodic blood tests to measure electrolytes, blood sugar and kidney function.

Some drugs used to treat high blood pressure act on the blood vessels, on the heart, or on the brain. *Propranolol* and other beta-blockers, as well as *methyldopa* and *hydralazine* are effective antihypertensive medications. Often, a combination of medications is given simultaneously. Each medication can have its own peculiar side effects. The main problem is the excessive lowering of the blood pressure, which will often lead to dizziness and faints. This can usually be reversed by decreasing the dosage.

Some diseases of the respiratory system, such as allergies,

do not always disappear as you grow older. *Antihistamines* are effective for burning eyes, itching nose, or mucus drip that often occurs with allergies. Although they may improve the symptoms, they may also cause excessive drowsiness and mental confusion and should not be taken if you are about to drive, and never when you drink alcohol.

Bronchodilators relieve the wheezing and shortness of breath that accompanies acute and chronic bronchitis or asthma. An infection of the bronchi or lungs aggravates these symptoms. Bronchodilators widen the bronchi and allow more air to reach the lungs. However, they sometimes lead to an excessively fast heartbeat, mental confusion, nausea, and vomiting. Usually an adjustment of dosage will alleviate these side effects.

An important class of drugs in this family is *theophylline,* which can be taken as pills, syrup, injection, and suppository. It is often prescribed in combination with the *beta-stimulators,* a group of medications that act like adrenaline. Among them are *isoproterenol, salbutamol, orciprenaline,* and *terbutaline.* They can be given as pills or as a "puffer," which is inhaled four or fives times a day. The preparations preferred for use in older people have less stimulatory effect on the heart than adrenaline itself.

For severe respiratory problems, *cortisone* may be required. There are many serious side effects from cortisone when taken orally or by injection, and its prolonged use should be avoided. Recently, a type of cortisone has been developed that can be inhaled, which reduces the usual side effects. A number of these preparations, such as *beclomethasone dipropionate,* can be taken through a "puffer" four or five times daily, often in conjunction with other bronchodilators.

Antibiotics are used for infections of the respiratory system as well as for infections in other parts of the body. The first group of drugs developed to counteract the growth and invasion of bacteria are the *sulphonamides,* which are not really antibiotics but are often called by this term. Some individuals develop a severe allergy to these preparations. If you are allergic to one kind of sulphonamide, you should not take any drug in this family.

Penicillin is also used to treat bacterial infections. Many medications in this family are manufactured synthetically and are effective against many types of bacteria. They are called *broad-spectrum* antibiotics. Most penicillins end in *cillin,* such as *ampicillin, cloxacillin,* and *amoxicillin.* In general, if you are allergic to one type of penicillin, you will be allergic to the others. Sometimes the allergy risk may have to be taken if the illness is severe and if a penicillin is the only drug available. However, precautions can be taken to avert a serious reaction. You should obtain a *Medic-Alert* bracelet that says you are allergic to penicillin, and always tell your doctor about allergies to antibiotics.

Another group of antibiotics closely related to the penicillins are the *cephalosporins,* also broad-spectrum antibiotics. People who are severely allergic to penicillin may also be allergic to these as well.

There are other types of antibiotics known as the *amino-glycosides,* including *streptomycin.* They are usually reserved for serious infections and the medication is given by injection. Another important group is *tetracycline,* also a broad-spectrum antibiotic which is used for less serious infections and is usually taken orally. This group can cause intestinal problems and may have to be stopped because of diarrhea. *Erythromycin* and *chloramphenicol* are older medications that inhibit certain types of bacteria. The latter must be used cautiously because it can cause a severe disorder of the bone marrow, although this is rare.

Antibiotics can be very effective in treating infections of the respiratory system, urinary tract, intestinal system, and heart. They should not be used indiscriminately, and they should never be taken without medical supervision.

Antacids, used to treat various gastrointestinal disorders, are usually sold without a prescription. In most individuals they have few serious side effects, although some cause diarrhea and others lead to constipation. It may be necessary to change the preparation depending on your reaction. The absorption of iron pills may be inhibited by the use of these substances, so they should not be taken together.

Laxatives and *stool softeners* are extremely popular among older individuals, and many become addicted to them because of chronic constipation. Whenever possible, it is better to discontinue the use of laxatives and replace them with a high-fiber diet. Sometimes stool softeners, such as *dioctyl sodium sulfosuccinate* or *psyllium mucilloid,* may be necessary to keep the bowels moving. *Milk of magnesia* and *lactulose* can also be effective. Avoid *mineral oil* for prolonged periods because it can interfere with the absorption of certain vitamins.

During the past few years, a new drug has become available which decreases the production of stomach acid. *Cimetidine* is the preparation presently available and it is effective in treating ulcers and is sometimes useful in the relief of symptoms from a hiatus hernia. It can cause mental confusion at times. *Metoclopramide* can be effective in the treatment of a hiatus hernia if severe symptoms are unrelieved by other medications. It can cause symptoms similar to Parkinson's disease in some people, however.

Antispasmodics are effective for abdominal cramps. Their major drawback is that they sometimes cause problems with the passage of urine.

Hormonal preparations are used to replace normal hormones that may be lacking. For instance, *thyroid hormone replacement* is necessary for the reversal of symptoms of hypothyroidism and *cortisone* is used to treat symptoms of Addison's disease, which is caused by insufficient cortisone in the body. Cortisone has other uses as well; it is used in much larger doses to control inflammation than when employed to reverse Addison's disease. *Female hormones* (estrogen) can be used to treat the symptoms of the menopause and can also prevent the progress and decrease the spread of cancer of the prostate gland in men. Hormone medications should be given with great discretion, and they should be closely supervised by a physician. Their potential for good is enormous, but they can have serious side effects if not watched carefully.

Anemia, a common problem in older individuals, has many causes. If it is due to a deficiency of *iron,* this may be prescribed as iron pills or injections. Iron should not be taken without a proper diagnosis of the cause of the anemia. If taken by mouth, the iron may make your stool very dark. Some people get diarrhea when they take iron, and others develop constipation. *Vitamin B_{12}* is used to treat pernicious anemia. It is effective for this disorder but should never be used as a "tonic." *Folic acid* is sometimes given to treat certain kinds of anemia. It has no side effects unless given inappropriately to a person who really needs vitamin B_{12}.

The drugs used in the treatment of malignant disease are too numerous to discuss. They change quickly, and usually an expert in cancer therapy (oncologist) must decide on the most appropriate drug for the specific disease. Because they are potent, they frequently have serious side effects and must be taken under close medical supervision.

There have been major strides in the treatment of Parkinson's disease recently. Drugs that contain *L-Dopa,* often combined with a substance that improves its results and decreases its side effects, are frequently prescribed. *Amantadine* is also used, as are some of the older *anticholinergic* drugs. These medications may be used in combination. The potential side effects include mental confusion or abnormal body movements. It is often necessary to alter the dosage periodically in order to achieve the optimal control of symptoms.

There has been a constant search for drugs that can be used to prevent strokes. *Anticoagulants* (blood thinners) are used for this purpose, as well as for the prevention and treatment of pulmonary emboli. In the early stages *heparin* is often given by injection and is frequently followed by treatment with *coumadin* anticoagulants orally. The main problem with these drugs is that they increase your risk of bleeding spontaneously or after an injury and this becomes enhanced with age. Therefore, if you are receiving anticoagulants, you must watch for blood in your urine or bowel movements and try to avoid physical injuries. These medications may have to be stopped if you require surgery. Blood tests are taken periodically to see if their dosage is correct.

The use of drugs to decrease the stickiness of blood has become very fashionable. It is hoped that they will prevent some people from having strokes. Among the medications are *aspirin, sulfinpyrazone,* and *dipyridamole,* which may be used in combination. They are also used to treat peripheral vascular disease because they may prevent further deterioration in the blood supply to the legs.

An important group of drugs that are often overused by older individuals are sleeping pills, or *hypnotics.* Sleep is a complex process, and whenever possible, sleep disorders should not be treated with these preparations. *Barbiturates* should not be used at all in older people. Many physicians prefer to use *chloral hydrate* instead. In recent years it has become popular to use *flurazepam,* and other preparations which are similar to diazepam, commonly used as a tranquilizer.

All the hypnotics are habit-forming. Because their effects diminish in time, the sleep disorder may become aggravated. It is more important to discover the cause for the sleep disturbance and deal with it at its source, rather than changing hypnotics or increasing their dosage. They all can cause mental confusion.

Medications for emotional disturbances are frequently prescribed for older people. The use of *minor tranquilizers,* such as diazepam, has reached almost epidemic proportions. Although they occasionally may be helpful, for the most part they are taken excessively. *Major tranquilizers* are used for serious mental illness or in cases of severe agitation. The most common drugs of this group are the *phenothiazines.* Although they have a calming effect, they sometimes increase mental symptoms, and they can cause or aggravate the symptoms of Parkinson's disease. They can also cause the blood pressure to fall, and some people develop abnormalities in liver function, which is reversible when the medication is stopped.

Antidepressant medications are beneficial for depressive illnesses, but they must be used with great discretion. Usually, a small dose is given and gradually increased in order to avoid side effects such as mental confusion and irregular heart rhythms. Some people complain of an excessively dry mouth, and this often occurs with phenothiazines as well.

Diabetes mellitus, a common ailment, improves with dietary changes. However, some people require *insulin.* This is more likely if the illness was acquired at an earlier age and if you are not overweight. The main problem with the use of insulin is excessive dosage, which may result in a hypoglycemic (low blood sugar) reaction. You will learn how to adjust your insulin dosage according to your diet and amount of exercise.

Some people benefit from *hypoglycemic* tablets, which increase the feeling of well-being and decrease the symptoms of diabetes. The two main families are the *sulphonylureas* and *biguanides. Chlorpropamide* and *tolbutamide* are examples of commonly used hypoglycemic pills. There has been controversy as to whether these medications should be used because some researchers think that they may increase the tendency to certain types of heart disease.

Your physician should not be expected to know the details of every medication, and he will frequently consult his desk references for information. You can help your physician by knowing your own medications. You should know the family to which they belong and the reason they were prescribed. If possible, you should know the generic name and the dosage. Review your medications periodically with your physician. It is your responsibility, as well as your physician's, to use medications accurately and carefully in order to obtain the maximum benefit.

CHAPTER 6

Diagnostic Tests

After your physician has taken a complete history of your illness and finished a physical examination, a number of tests may be necessary to make a diagnosis. Even though many minor illnesses and some more serious ones can be diagnosed on the basis of the interview and physical examination alone, most require further investigation to confirm the nature of the illness or evaluate your response to treatment.

For instance, it may be clear that you are suffering from angina pectoris after you tell your physician that you get chest pain when you walk, but it is relieved when you rest. You may even have tried a friend's nitroglycerin tablets and found that they relieved your discomfort. The diagnosis is almost certain from this information alone. During the physical examination your physician may find evidence of atherosclerosis because your blood vessels show evidence of narrowing. This would increase the likelihood of the symptoms being the result of angina pectoris.

Although medication can be prescribed on the basis of this

information alone, most physicians will do an *electrocardiogram,* or ECG, to see if any damage to the heart has occurred. An ECG is also a useful record for comparison should you suffer from a heart attack at a later date. Various blood tests are also important to try to discover if any factors might increase your risk of a heart attack. Other tests can help your physician decide on medication dosages. X-rays would also be useful to determine if there are any complications and for comparison should your symptoms get worse.

Whenever tests are done, the physician should consider the possible benefit, its cost to you or to the medical system that covers you, and the relative dangers of the procedure. In some medical systems cost is not a great factor, and in others it is. We would all like to believe that "no expense will be spared" for our health, but this is not the case even under "socialized" medicine. In one way or the other we all pay the costs, and physicians should consider these factors when they order tests.

As you grow older, you may have more than one condition at the same time, and more tests may be necessary to make a diagnosis or to follow the results of treatment than in younger people. Some tests measure the amounts of various substances in your blood, urine, sputum, and spinal fluid. For the most part these tests have little danger. Although taking blood may be uncomfortable, it is rare that even after many tests you will suffer from the blood loss. To get fluid from the lungs, for instance, or fluid that surrounds the spinal cord, a needle must be inserted deeper into the body. Although there is little danger with these procedures, they are slightly more risky than blood tests. However, the diseases for which these tests are done are usually more dangerous, so the need for the test is greater than the risk.

Other tests depend on *X-rays* and more modern procedures, such as *nuclear scans* and *computerized scans (CAT scans).* They allow the physicians to "see into" the body without surgery. These examinations that rely on small amounts of radiation and the *echograms,* which depend on sound waves, help physicians diagnose internal problems with relatively little danger to their patients. The cost of diagnostic tests is great, but the information they provide can be very important. In every case the risk of the test must be weighed against the benefits of making a diagnosis and the danger of not treating the illness.

With modern technology, instruments have been developed that can pass through the body openings such as the mouth and anus to internal organs without surgery. These low-risk procedures, called *endoscopy*, require a highly trained physician and are often done only in hospitals or specially equipped clinics.

A *biopsy*, to analyze a sample of diseased tissue, may be needed to make an accurate diagnosis. Many illnesses look alike, and sometimes the test results may be the same for different illnesses, for which the treatment may be completely opposite. Biopsies are somewhat more dangerous than other diagnostic tests, but they are usually reserved for more severe illnesses. Sometimes more than one biopsy may be necessary, either to make a diagnosis or to follow the results of treatment. Many people think that biopsies are used only to diagnose malignancies and become unnecessarily worried when a biopsy is proposed. A biopsy may be necessary to diagnose many other illnesses including infection and inflammation.

Another important group of tests are those that measure electrical activity in the heart, brain, nerves, and muscles, all of which have various electrical properties. The tests, which are usually without danger but require highly skilled technical and medical personnel, may be used to diagnose either common or obscure illnesses and to follow the outcome of treatment.

When you go to your physician, you should expect that some type of diagnostic test will be done. In most instances the tests will be simple. If you have a more complicated illness, the tests may be more involved. If you are hospitalized, you will probably have many more tests. It is quite reasonable to ask your physician for an outline and explanation of the tests that he will do. If you trust your physician, you should allow him to do the simple tests without giving an elaborate explanation, however. Certain tests, such as biopsies, require your consent to ensure that you understand the risk involved. If you have had many tests and it seems that your illness is not improving, you or your family should ask your doctor for an explanation.

Many older people feel that they are used as "guinea pigs" when tests are done. This is partly because they do not understand the tests and perhaps they are suspicious that they will not be treated with the same respect as younger people. However, it is highly unlikely that any tests will be done that have not been proven to be safe and effective. Even though a test may not give definitive information, the fact that it is normal is also important for the physician to know. You are not being experimented on when you have these tests. Ask why they are being done if you are uncertain. You have a right to know.

BLOOD TESTS

Usually, your physician will request blood tests because almost all illnesses cause some abnormality in the constituents of the blood. Blood tests are often the easiest way to determine that you have a disorder. They are easy to do, have no danger, and if done carefully usually cause little discomfort. They can be repeated readily to obtain diagnostic information and measure the results of treatment.

Blood consists of a fluid called *plasma*, which carries red and white blood cells. Red cells, or *erythrocytes*, carry oxygen and carbon dioxide. They contain a special chemical substance called *hemoglobin*, which allows oxygen and carbon dioxide to enter or leave the cell. In many diseases the ability of the body to keep up the normal level of red cells and hemoglobin is disturbed. This is determined by a *blood count*, which tells the physician if the red cells and hemoglobin are normal. If they are too low, the condition is called *anemia*.

There are a number of varieties of white blood cells, or *leucocytes,* which help the body fight infection. In certain illnesses there may be either too many or too few white blood cells, or the ones produced may be abnormal. If you have too many white blood cells, you may have an infection, which stimulates the body to fight the germs. On the other hand, a disorder of the white blood cells may make you more susceptible to infection.

Another important component of the blood is the *platelets,* small cell-like particles that induce blood clotting when an artery or vein is injured. However, there may be too many or too few platelets in certain disorders. This can make the blood too sticky, which causes blood clots to form within blood vessels, or it can keep the blood from clotting normally and increase your tendency to bleed.

All the blood cells and platelets are produced in the *bone marrow,* found within the bones of the body. This is the "factory" that manufactures blood cells and allows them to enter the bloodstream according to the needs of the body. Sometimes the bone marrow becomes diseased and produces excess amounts of blood cells or too few of its components. This results in various blood diseases.

The blood cells are carried in the plasma, which also contains many other components that are vital for the normal, healthy function of the body. *Hormones,* produced by glands, are also transported by the plasma, as are *salts,* which keep the body environment normal. All *nutrients* from food pass into the plasma from the gastrointestinal tract and are circulated throughout the body. *Antibodies,* which are produced to fight disease, all *medications,* and the *byproducts of metabolism* are contained in the plasma.

As medicine progresses, we learn more and more about changes that occur within the components of the blood. Therefore, the number and complexity of blood tests has grown enormously in the past few years. The elements in the blood that can be affected by medications, either by design or unintentionally as side effects, can also be determined.

Ask your physician what tests are being done. He may tell you their chemical name or that he is examining your "kidneys" or "liver." Sometimes blood tests are repeated, and you may wonder why. Many older people complain that their blood is being taken too often, but it is often advisable to repeat blood tests in order to make a diagnosis and to see the outcome of treatment. If tests are reordered, ask your physician why. In many instances it is more important for the physician to know about the *changes* that occur in the blood than to see the results of a single measurement.

The following is a summary of the most common blood tests, but new tests are always being discovered. Tests are done by commercial and hospital laboratories, but ones that require special equipment or expertise may be sent elsewhere. Before you leave your physician, ask how you will find out about the results of the tests. Ask whether he will want to see you again to discuss the tests or whether he can tell you the results over the telephone. A physician will usually tell you that if the tests are normal, you will not hear from him and know that "no news is good news." If you have gone to a specialist for the tests, he may tell your physician the results. Make sure that you know what was done and who has the answers so that unnecessary duplication is avoided.

SERUM ELECTROLYTE TESTS

Blood contains various salts that are needed for normal function. The electrolytes can be affected by high blood pressure, diabetes mellitus, and heart failure, as well as by many of the medications used for their treatment. If you are receiving diuretics (water pills) for one of these conditions, you should expect to have your electrolytes measured every few months. This is necessary to avoid side effects.

BUN (BLOOD UREA NITROGEN) AND CREATININE TESTS

BUN and creatinine are normal waste products produced by the body. Under ordinary conditions they are removed from the blood by the kidneys. In a disease of the kidneys these elements accumulate, however. Kidney disease and high blood pressure are closely interrelated. It is important to have these substances measured if you suffer from high blood pressure as well. Medications used to treat heart disease, kidney disorders, and high blood pressure include diuretics and digoxin. The level of BUN and creatinine in the blood will determine their dosage. If the kidney disease becomes severe, the level of BUN and creatinine rises. During tests of kidney function, the electrolytes are often measured at the same time.

LIVER FUNCTION TESTS

The liver, the main factory of the body, manufactures important substances from nutrients. The liver also disposes of the waste products of metabolism. *Bile,* produced by the liver, is necessary for the digestion of fats. Therefore, liver abnormalities can have a severe effect on the body.

Liver tests also examine *enzymes,* which are contained within liver cells. These leak into or accumulate in the blood when the organ is damaged or diseased. An excess amount of *bilirubin* in the blood may indicate a blockage of the biliary ducts, which allow bile to flow from the liver to the small intestine. When this accumulates, a yellow discoloration of the skin *(jaundice)* usually occurs.

The severity of liver diseases varies, so it is often necessary for function tests to be taken frequently during a liver illness. As the disease subsides, your physician may continue to measure these substances to assure that the liver has returned to normal. In some disorders, the symptoms may be very mild. Sometimes the only abnormality that may confirm that an illness is present is a mild irregularity in liver function tests, so these would be done periodically to judge whether the disease is progressing or resolving.

URIC ACID TESTS

Uric acid is a normal constituent of the blood. If it accumulates, it can cause kidney damage or gout, a painful condition of the joints. People who suffer from gout usually have raised amounts of uric acid. Kidney disease and diuretics used to treat high blood pressure and heart failure can increase the level of uric acid in the blood.

If you suffer from gout or have a raised uric acid level as a result of kidney disease or the use of medications, your blood should be checked periodically. This is important because there are now effective medications that lower the amount of uric acid. Periodic blood tests confirm that the drugs are working.

CALCIUM AND PHOSPHORUS TESTS

Calcium and phosphorus are usually measured together because they interact with each other very closely. They are affected by diseases of the bones and kidneys and when the parathyroid glands are abnormal. Certain medications also affect their blood levels. The tests may be repeated if you suffer from an illness that alters their normal values.

THYROID FUNCTION TESTS

Disease of the thyroid gland is quite common in older individuals, but the diagnosis is less easily made than in younger people. Physicians often order thyroid function tests to look for evidence of excessive or decreased working of the gland. If you have thyroid disease and have been treated for it or are presently taking thyroid medications, you can expect to have your thyroid tests measured periodically.

HORMONE TESTS

In addition to thyroid, hormones produced by other endocrine glands can be measured to determine whether these glands are working normally. When the body produces an excess or too little of an individual hormone an illness ensues. Measurement of the amount of hormone in the blood can help diagnose these disorders and evaluate treatment.

BLOOD SUGAR TESTS

Abnormalities of blood sugar control are found in diabetes mellitus, so it is important that your blood sugar be tested to diagnose the disorder and to follow its control once treatment has started. If you are suspected of having diabetes mellitus, it may be sufficient to have an isolated sample of blood sugar measured. If this is excessively high, a definite diagnosis sometimes can be made. Often it is better to have the level of blood sugar estimated while you are in a fasting state (without breakfast). At other times, a measurement done two hours after a meal is more useful.

If diabetes mellitus cannot be diagnosed from a fasting sugar sample or one taken two hours after a meal, your physician may request a *glucose tolerance test*, in which you drink a measured amount of liquid sugar. An estimation of your blood sugar level is done before you drink the liquid and tests are repeated for the next few hours. This determines whether the amount of blood sugar is excessively high.

If you are being treated for diabetes mellitus, you must have your sugar levels measured periodically. The blood may be taken when you are in a fasting state, or after a meal, or in the afternoon, depending on whether you are taking pills, insulin, or merely following a diabetic diet.

ERYTHROCYTE SEDIMENTATION RATE (ESR) TESTS

The ESR has been available for many years, and even though we still do not completely understand how it works, it is very useful. The sedimentation rate becomes elevated when the body is suffering from an inflammatory illness. Its main use is in arthritic diseases, but it is also used in some blood disorders. It may also be helpful in alerting the physician to an arthritic, inflammatory or blood disorder and in assessing the results of treatment. Therefore, the ESR may be measured frequently if you are being treated for an inflammatory or arthritic condition.

ARTHRITIS TESTS

In addition to the sedimentation rate, special tests can be used to diagnose the various types of arthritis. For instance, rheumatoid arthritis may be characterized by the *rheumatoid factor*, which is an abnormal antibody found in the blood of people with this disorder. With treatment, the level of this substance in the blood may decrease, confirming that the therapy is effective. There are many other types of tests for arthritic disorders. Depending on the particular type of arthritic problem, your physician will request the appropriate test.

URINE TESTS

Urine, which is produced by the kidneys, contains a large amount of water, within which the body's waste products are dissolved. Infections that occur in the urinary system can lead to abnormalities in the urine. If the kidneys are damaged, the normal amounts of elements in the urine are altered. During illnesses such as diabetes mellitus, sugar may "leak" into the urine. Its measurement can be useful in controlling the degree of blood sugar elevation.

Some urine tests require *any* sample of urine. A cup or two is usually sufficient for many of the simple tests. Other tests require a whole day's urine, sometimes collected in a special container that contains a preservative to keep it from decomposing. It is sometimes necessary to bring urine that has been passed the first thing in the morning.

When the physician checks your urine for infection, it is important that it be collected in a way that keeps the bacteria in the urine from being contaminated by the bacteria on your skin. This urine is collected as a *midstream specimen (MSU)* or *clean-catch* urine. Such a sample requires a sterile container so that only the germs in the urine are examined.

In men it is usually easier to collect a clean-catch specimen. It is often only necessary for a man to urinate into the toilet, and while the stream is flowing to put the sterile jar or cup under it without interrupting the flow. It is like filling a cup with water from a running tap.

In women it is a little more complicated because many bacteria normally inhabit the area around the female urethra. If these enter the container with the urine, there may be evidence of an infection that is not really from the urine or kidneys. It is therefore necessary for women to clean the area around the urethra and vagina with sterile water before collecting the urine. Then, as the urine flows, while standing over a toilet, the specimen is collected in a sterile container without interrupting the stream. In older women it may be necessary to get the help of a technician or nurse for the specimen to be obtained accurately.

SPINAL FLUID AND RELATED TESTS

In addition to blood and urine, other fluids can provide important information. To get a sample of these fluids, a needle is inserted to extract the fluid. Although there is little danger from the procedure, it may be more uncomfortable than the sampling of blood or urine.

The brain and spinal cord are surrounded by *spinal fluid*, which acts as a protective cushion for the nervous system. In health the fluid is clear and contains normal amounts of salts, nutrients, and a few white blood cells for protection. During illnesses in which the nervous system is damaged, the spinal fluid may develop abnormalities that make it possible to diagnose the disorder.

To obtain spinal fluid, a thin needle is passed into the spinal canal through the lower part of the back. This test is called a *lumbar puncture* (spinal tap). While the needle is in the spinal canal, the pressure of the spinal fluid can also be measured. The fluid is extracted and analyzed to see if there are any infections or bleeding within the nervous system. Some special tests require that substances be injected into the spinal canal. In certain infections antibiotics are introduced through the needle into the spinal fluid. It is occasionally necessary to repeat the lumbar puncture in order to follow the effects of treatment.

Sometimes fluid accumulates in the pleural space around the lungs or in the abdomen, and very occasionally around the heart. At times there may be excess fluid within a joint. Whenever there is an abnormal collection of fluid in the body, it may be necessary to extract it for analysis. Obtaining the fluid may also result in an improvement in symptoms, as when it is taken from around the heart or lungs. Usually a small amount of local anesthetic is used to freeze the skin and muscles before the needle is inserted. Although you may feel the pressure of the needle, you should not experience an undue amount of pain.

BACTERIOLOGICAL CULTURES

During infections a sample of the infected material is analyzed to determine which bacterium or virus is responsible. The material is sent to the laboratory for *culture*. This allows the bacteria or viruses to grow on special substances so that they can be identified. Also, they can be tested against various antibiotics, which helps the physician decide which treatment will be most effective.

One of the most common substances that is sent for culture is sputum (phlegm) during infections of the respiratory tract. It is obtained by having you cough the phlegm into a sterile container. Sometimes samples are obtained through a fine plastic tube that is passed into the trachea and the sputum is suctioned into a test tube. An examination of an infected sample of sputum allows the physician to choose the correct antibiotic for treatment. This is especially important in older individuals, who have less tolerance for infections.

Because infections of the urinary tract are common in older people, urine samples are often needed for bacteriological examination. Wounds that contain pus are sampled to see which bacteria are causing the infections. In serious infections there may be bacteria in the blood (septicemia), so the physician may take blood cultures to identify the bacteria. The same procedure is necessary if you are suspected of suffering from bacterial endocarditis. The blood is collected in special sterilized bottles that contain a kind of soup in which bacteria will grow. It is no more painful than a standard blood test.

Samples of fluid are usually sent for culture, as well as for other tests, so the physician can determine whether the disorder is caused by an infection, which would require treatment with antibiotics. The results of cultures take a few days for most bacteria, but special bacteria, such as tuberculosis, may take many weeks before the results are known. Viruses are much more difficult to culture, and they also often take weeks before accurate answers are obtained.

X-RAYS

Most people at some time in their lives have had an X-ray. X-rays produce images of the body and allow physicians to see what is happening within the abdomen, chest, bones, and skull. They permit the diagnosis of different kinds of illnesses, and some may have to be repeated in order to follow the results of treatment.

In the past little attention was paid to the amount of radiation that patients were exposed to during X-ray procedures. It took years before it became clear that there was a potential danger from excessive radiation. Technical advances have reduced the amount of radiation, and measures can be taken to decrease the amount of exposure that is received by parts of the body that should be protected from radiation.

The question is often raised about whether the danger of X-rays is greater than that of the illness for which they are being done. In children and in young adults there is no doubt that it is important to minimize the amount of radiation. In older people the danger seems to be less pronounced because birth defects are not an issue.

Whether or not X-rays cause cancer in older people is still not completely clear. If X-rays are done carefully and with proper supervision, they do not appear to pose a particular threat to the health of the older person. In most cases any danger from the X-ray is outweighed by the beneficial information that is obtained.

Some X-rays have no real danger other than that related to the amount of radiation received. Other X-rays require special chemical substances that are either swallowed or injected, and they may have a degree of hazard, especially in the older person. Even if the risk is not particularly great, some X-rays require preparation that can be uncomfortable and difficult for older individuals. These factors must be taken into account before an X-ray is ordered. Sometimes physicians modify the procedure to make it easier for the older person. If you had a difficult time with an X-ray procedure in the past and your physician orders a similar X-ray again, let him know so that appropriate steps can be taken to avoid discomfort and danger.

PLAIN X-RAYS

No preparation is necessary for plain X-rays, and other than the small amounts of radiation, there is no risk. They usually can be repeated as often as necessary. The most common X-rays are those of the chest, spine, bones, skull, and abdomen.

You may wonder why your physician is repeating X-rays. An X-ray is not only useful to make a diagnosis but also may be necessary to follow the outcome of treatment. For example, a chest X-ray, probably the most common, gives a picture of the heart and lungs. It can be used to diagnose heart failure or pneumonia and will probably be repeated on a number of occasions to make sure that the therapy has been successful.

CONTRAST X-RAYS

Contrast X-rays require that a chemical substance be swallowed, injected, or given as an enema. The substances used for the "contrast" appear on the X-ray and leave the body after it is finished. They usually do not have any side effects, unless for some unusual reason you are allergic to iodine, which is contained in some of these substances. If you have had a reaction to iodine during an X-ray procedure in the past, inform your physician whenever an X-ray is ordered.

BARIUM X-RAYS, G. I. SERIES, AND BARIUM ENEMA

Barium, a white, sticky substance, is often used to investigate disorders of the gastrointestinal tract, such as ulcer disease, hiatus hernia, benign and malignant tumors, and inflammatory disorders of the bowel. It can be swallowed to outline the esophagus, stomach, and small intestine or given as an enema if the lower intestine is to be examined.

The *G. I. series (upper gastrointestinal series),* or *barium swallow,* is used to diagnose diseases of the esophagus, stomach, and small intestine. The barium, which tastes chalky but is usually flavored to make it palatable, can cause some constipation, and you will probably be given a laxative to help you expel it.

The test is usually done with a fluoroscope or television device, which allows the physician to watch the barium flow into the esophagus and stomach. A barium swallow is done in the fasting state. Any food or fluid that has been taken in the eight or ten hours before the study may interfere with an accurate interpretation of the X-rays.

A *barium enema* uses the same substance, but it is inserted into the rectum. This X-ray is used to examine the lower intestine (large bowel). The test and the preparation for it are somewhat uncomfortable. Usually it is necessary to take laxatives for a day or two prior to the X-ray to be certain that the bowel is clear. I sometimes recommend a more gradual preparation with a fluid diet for a day or two before. This often avoids the need for strong laxatives.

GALLBLADDER X-RAYS

Gallbladder disorders are quite common in older people, but X-ray abnormalities are found more frequently than the actual illnesses that they may produce. Sometimes a gallstone is found in an older individual who has no symptoms of gallbladder disease. These routine X-rays show the gallbladder and the biliary ducts, and the connection to the small intestine (see page 258).

The simplest type of gallbladder X-ray, the *oral cholecystogram,* requires that you swallow a number of tablets that contain an iodine substance that accumulates in the gallbladder. The X-ray is taken the morning after the tablets are swallowed. You may be given a fatty food snack in the middle of the X-ray to see if the gallbladder expels its contents normally. Any gallstones would also be shown in this study. The tablets can cause a few loose bowel movements on the day of the examination.

A second type of gallbladder X-ray is the *intravenous cholangiogram,* which consists of an iodine-containing fluid being injected into a vein. The fluid is concentrated by the liver and passes into the biliary ducts. There it outlines the tubes that connect the gallbladder and liver to the intestines. A blockage to the outflow of bile may appear on this X-ray if it is done early in the disease. Other than the problem of allergy to iodine, these X-rays have no danger.

A *transhepatic cholangiogram,* the third type of X-ray, may be used in more severe gallbladder diseases or when a physician suspects a prolonged blockage to the outflow of bile. This X-ray is usually done in anticipation of surgery to relieve the obstruction. If there is a complete blockage, you may require surgery fairly urgently. A very fine needle injecting an iodine dye is inserted into the liver. The dye enters a bile "pool" and then flows into the biliary ducts. The risk is slightly greater than other X-rays but much smaller than the illness for which it is being done.

KIDNEY X-RAYS

The most common X-ray to investigate kidney disorders and diseases of the urinary tract is an *intravenous pyelogram* (usually called IVP). This is similar to an intravenous cholangiogram. An iodine-containing substance is injected into a vein and the kidneys are outlined by the dye as it enters the urine. An enema to clear the bowel is usually required prior to the test. This X-ray cannot be done if you are allergic to iodine.

ANGIOGRAPHY

Angiography is a relatively new development in the field of radiology. An *angiogram* is an X-ray taken while an iodine substance is injected into blood vessels. This reveals any abnormalities in the organs that they supply. Angiography can be used to visualize the blood supply of every organ in the body. With little danger, many hidden parts of the body can be outlined by the pattern of the blood vessels. Diagnoses that were previously elusive are more easily made with the assistance of these X-rays.

Angiograms are done of the *carotid* blood vessels (blood vessels to the brain) in patients suffering from strokes. They may show the reason for the stroke and may help determine if treatment can relieve symptoms or prevent further strokes. In addition, other abnormalities of the brain can be shown with a *cerebral (brain) angiogram,* such as benign or malignant tumors and blood clots (hematoma), which occasionally press on the brain. Clots may be found in older people who have suffered a fall.

A *peripheral angiogram* is done to see whether there is a blockage in the blood vessels to the legs. A vascular (blood vessel) surgeon might be able to bypass such a blockage or remove a clot that has formed.

An *abdominal angiogram* outlines the arteries and veins that supply the large and small bowel. Occasionally, older people bleed from various parts of the bowel, and this may not show up on barium X-rays. In these cases an abdominal angiogram may demonstrate the area of hemorrhage and the exact site of blood loss, especially if done at the time of active bleeding.

A *cardiac (heart) angiogram* shows the blood vessels supplying the heart. This is performed in patients who have angina pectoris or who have had heart attacks (myocardial infarction), if the physician is considering a bypass operation to increase the heart's blood supply.

All angiograms have a small degree of risk. The main danger is bleeding from the site of insertion of the thin plastic tube (catheter) that is used to inject the dye. Blockage of the blood vessel, which occurs very rarely, usually means that the underlying disease is severe. In most cases the minimal risk of the angiogram is less than the danger of the disease. I have recommended these tests to many elderly patients and have rarely observed serious side effects.

NUCLEAR SCANS, ECHOGRAMS, AND CAT SCANS

Many technical marvels developed in the past twenty years allow physicians to examine the internal organs without having to perform surgery. Nuclear scans, echograms, and CAT scans provide physicians with valuable knowledge, and with virtually no danger and little discomfort to you.

NUCLEAR-MEDICINE SCANS

This relatively new method uses extremely small doses of radioactive substances to outline various organs. The amount of radioactive material is minute, however. Thus far, nothing suggests that there is any danger of this radioactive material causing cancer or other side effects. The personnel working with these substances, who are exposed to far greater doses for longer periods, have not been shown to suffer from cumulative effects of the radiation if it is used carefully.

The word *nuclear* unfortunately often brings up the fear of cancer. I have seen older people become absolutely terrified that they have cancer because they were sent for a nuclear scan. They confuse *radioactive scans* with *radiation therapy*, which is used to treat cancer. It is very important to ask the reason for these tests so that you can feel assured that they do not mean that you are suffering from a malignant disease. Although these tests may be used to diagnose cancer, they are extremely useful and important in determining countless other noncancerous diseases.

The wonderful thing about nuclear scans is that, with virtually no danger or discomfort, they provide information that is not easily obtainable through X-rays or other tests. This means that the scans can be repeated, not only for the purpose of diagnosis but also to follow the results of treatment.

A very small amount of radioactive substance is injected into a vein and is carried to the organ that is being examined. Measurements of the amount of radiation in the organ show how it is working. The most important scans are *brain scans,* often used to diagnose strokes, and *lung scans,* frequently requested when there is a suspicion of a *pulmonary embolus* (blood clot to the lungs). *Bone scans* can help diagnose obscure disorders of the skeleton. There are also scans of the thyroid gland, liver and biliary tree, kidneys, lymph nodes, bone marrow, blood vessels, and heart. These studies are often done in conjunction with other investigations, such as X-rays and echograms.

ECHOGRAMS

Echograms use sound waves, which are directed through the body and reflect what is happening in various organs. It is a fairly new application of a technique that has been known for many years. There is no known danger from these tests; sound waves do not seem to cause any disorders in the human body. Therefore, the tests can be repeated as often as necessary.

Echograms can discern small abnormalities within the abdomen, heart, and pelvis. When used in conjunction with X-rays and nuclear scans, they may allow a diagnosis without surgery.

CAT SCANS

The CAT scan (computerized axial tomography) is a recent, major technological advance in the field of X-rays. It allows many rapid X-rays to be taken simultaneously at slightly different angles and different points of focus. The end result is a three-dimensional picture of any part of the body. The first use of CAT scans was on the brain. Many elusive problems are diagnosed much more easily and with less danger or discomfort than with plain X-rays, arteriograms, nuclear scans, and echograms. Often the CAT scan is so accurate that other tests can be avoided.

Abdominal CAT scans investigate diseases of the abdomen, liver and spleen, kidneys, and the deep spaces within the abdominal cavity. The abdominal CAT scan has not replaced the other X-ray procedures, but it greatly adds to the ability to make elusive diagnoses. CAT scans are also used for the chest and spinal canal.

The equipment used for these scans is enormously expensive, and the cost eventually is paid by all of us who use the health care system. Ultimately, CAT scans may prove to be a relatively less expensive and more effective way of investigating many illnesses. However, it must be left to the discretion of the physician to order a CAT scan. In some places patients and their families appear to be requesting these tests as a way of assuring themselves that they are not suffering from a serious disease. No single test can do that.

ENDOSCOPY

To understand the nature of many disorders, physicians often have a "peek" inside through the openings into the body. For many years the parts of the body that could be examined with ease were the mouth, nose, throat, and anus. With technological advances it has become easier and less uncomfortable for physicians to insert highly sensitive instruments along these passages. The instruments are called by the name of the orifice that they enter. The procedure is called by the same name and ends in the suffix *scopy*. For example, sigmoidoscopy means *looking into* the lower part of the bowel.

Easier tests may be done by any physician; others are so sophisticated that only a specialist would have the skill to do the test properly. They have virtually no danger, although some of them are uncomfortable. Many can be done in a doctor's office and some on an out-patient basis in a hospital, which does not require an overnight stay.

SIGMOIDOSCOPY

Sigmoidoscopy is one of the oldest investigations of this type. A rigid metal or plastic tube is inserted through the anus into the lower large bowel. (A shorter instrument, called a *proctoscope*, is sometimes used if only the anus and lower part of the rectum are to be examined.) The tube is lubricated to allow it to move easily into the intestine. You may be asked to lie on your side or to support yourself on your elbows with your buttocks in the air. Although the test is somewhat uncomfortable, it can usually be done by a family doctor or internist, as well as by a specialist.

The diagnosis of inflammation and tumors of the large intestine can often be made from this test. Many physicians recommend that an older person have this done at least once a year. In conjunction with a chemical test of the stool for blood and a rectal examination, this is an important step in diagnosing the earliest signs of disease of the large bowel.

COLONOSCOPY

Colonoscopy is possible because of the recent development of *fiber optics.* Flexible glass fibers transmit light over great distances at all angles. If the fiberglass is enclosed in a telescopelike instrument, it can be passed into the lower bowel to examine the whole large intestine. Whereas the sigmoidoscope is a rigid instrument, the *colonoscope* is flexible.

If you are being examined for anemia or bleeding from the large bowel and an answer has not been found, *colonoscopy* may be necessary. Sometimes small tumors that are seen on a barium enema can be removed through the instrument without the need for surgery. At other times, a barium X-ray may not reveal a tumor that is subsequently seen during colonoscopy. The test, which takes anywhere from forty-five minutes to an hour and a half, requires that you have your bowel well cleaned with laxatives and enemas beforehand. It is somewhat uncomfortable, but it can be done in most people regardless of age. Usually, a gastroenterologist or a surgeon specializing in diseases of the bowel will perform the test.

GASTROSCOPY

Gastroscopy is similar to colonoscopy, and the instrument used is almost identical. It is passed through the mouth into the esophagus and stomach. The physician may be able to determine the cause of bleeding from the upper intestine or see if there is obstruction to the passage of food. If something abnormal appears on a barium swallow, the gastroscopy may allow a specific diagnosis to be made without the need for abdominal surgery.

This procedure is done in the fasting state. Usually, the mouth and the back of the throat is "frozen" with a local anesthetic. Many physicians use small doses of tranquilizers to make you feel less tense during the examination. This test should not be omitted on the basis of age alone. It can be done even on the very ill, and it may make the difference between an accurate and a "presumptive" diagnosis.

A full investigation of the gastrointestinal tract may include a rectal examination followed by a sigmoidoscopy and perhaps a barium enema and barium swallow. Colonoscopy and gastroscopy may be required if the diagnosis is elusive. A set of gallbladder X-rays may also be needed to make sure that symptoms are not coming from the biliary tree, rather than from the intestines.

BRONCHOSCOPY

To diagnose diseases of the bronchi and lungs, it is sometimes necessary to look into the respiratory system rather than rely on X-rays alone. A *bronchoscope* is a thin, flexible instrument that can be passed through the nose or mouth into the trachea and down the bronchi. During the examination you will probably receive a local anesthetic and a mild tranquilizer. Samples of sputum can be obtained during the test, and tumors or other abnormalities can be seen and samples or biopsies taken.

CYSTOSCOPY

The urinary tract can be investigated through X-rays (IVP) and echograms and by urine tests. A *cystoscopy* may be done if there is bleeding from the urinary tract or difficulty with the passage of urine. It is more commonly necessary for men because of disorders of the prostate gland. A local anesthetic can be used, although it is frequently carried out under a general anesthetic. The procedure, which is somewhat uncomfortable, takes only ten or fifteen minutes and may have to be repeated. It is often possible to remove small tumors that grow in the bladder through the cystoscope, which means that surgery may be avoided.

BIOPSIES

Many illnesses appear to be similar and yet are quite different in terms of their ultimate outcome and treatment. Often, despite many tests of body fluids and innumerable X-rays and scans, a definite explanation of a disease is not clear. Under these circumstances a *biopsy* may be necessary to define its exact nature.

In a biopsy a small piece of the diseased tissue is removed and examined under a microscope. The specimen may also be sent for special biochemical studies, as well as for culture. In most instances there is at least a mild degree of discomfort, and sometimes there may be a small risk. This depends on the type of biopsy and how it is obtained. For instance, a biopsy of the skin has less hazard than a biopsy of the liver, which lies within the abdominal cavity. Often, a biopsy will make a great difference in the ability of the physician to treat you effectively. Unless it will add to your well-being, a biopsy will not be requested unless it is absolutely necessary. If you are confronted with a biopsy, ask your physician why and what the likely complications might be.

BONE MARROW BIOPSY

A *bone marrow* test is not always considered a biopsy, but in fact it is. The blood cells are made in the bone marrow and enter the bloodstream. A bone marrow specimen shows the younger varieties of blood cells. It is not always possible to diagnose disorders of the blood by blood tests alone.

An area of bone, either in the breastbone (sternum) or in a pelvic bone, is anesthetized with a local injection. A needle is then inserted into the bone and a sample of the bone marrow removed. The procedure takes about ten minutes and usually causes relatively little discomfort and has virtually no danger.

LUNG BIOPSY

A biopsy of the pleura (lining of the chest wall) or lung may be necessary if you have a disorder of the respiratory system that cannot be determined by X-rays and an examination of your sputum. If fluid collects in the pleural space, it is not possible to tell its cause without obtaining a sample of the liquid, because a number of illnesses can affect the pleural fluid in the same way.

A disease can affect the lung without causing fluid to collect. It may be necessary to do a *bronchoscopy,* which allows the physician to see any abnormalities within the bronchi. If something unexpected is seen, it is often possible to take a biopsy through the bronchoscope. However, the abnormal process may be out of reach of the bronchoscope, in which case a needle is inserted through the skin of the chest wall into the lung. This is called a *needle lung biopsy,* and it is not always

135

successful in obtaining the tissue. Therefore, an *open lung biopsy* may be necessary. This involves making a small cut through the chest wall and removing a tiny piece of lung. After this type of procedure a tube may be placed in the chest for a few hours to keep the lung expanded until the hole closes. Although more complex than the other biopsies, in almost all cases it can be done without danger. It is considered only when the diagnosis is elusive.

LIVER BIOPSY

The liver can be affected by many diseases that may have similar abnormal liver function tests and nuclear scans. A *liver biopsy* often permits a definite diagnosis. Some liver diseases improve quickly and others linger and may require more potent medications. So more than one biopsy may be done during the course of an illness and treatment.

Invariably, the seriousness of the disease warrants the small hazard involved. The skin of the upper abdomen is frozen with a local anesthetic. You will then be instructed to hold your breath as a fine needle is quickly put into your liver and withdrawn with the specimen. The test takes only a few moments and causes little discomfort. In rare instances there is some bleeding after the test, but this usually stops quickly. It is extremely rare for there to be any dangerous effects of this examination.

MUSCLE AND SKIN BIOPSIES

Muscle and *skin biopsies* can also be done. Small tumors of the skin are often removed at the time of biopsy. Many conditions affect the cells or the blood vessels of the muscles. Some neurological diseases that affect the muscles can be determined through a biopsy. The procedure is simple and can often be done within a few minutes. The muscles of the thigh or upper arm are common sites of the biopsy, and no danger is involved.

A number of unusual illnesses that mainly affect the elderly can cause damage to blood vessels. A biopsy of a *blood vessel* may clarify a diagnosis. One of the common disorders is *polymyalgia rheumatica*, a strange disease that causes unusual aches and pains. A biopsy of a small artery in the scalp may be necessary. The test takes a few moments and has no danger. An accurate diagnosis In this case is essential, because lack of proper treatment can result in blindness.

ELECTROCARDIOGRAM (ECG)

Heart function can be evaluated in a number of ways. A physical examination and a chest X-ray are crucial. However, different types of *electrocardiograms* give information that cannot be obtained by any other means.

A special kind of muscle in the heart receives its stimulation from an electrical system that governs how the heart beats. An electrocardio*graph* records the contraction of the muscle and the electrical impulses. By studying the ECG (or EKG) patterns and changes, physicians can diagnose many heart disorders.

An ordinary electrocardiogram takes about five minutes and is completely painless and has absolutely no danger. It is done either routinely in order to have a record for future reference or at the time of a suspected heart disturbance. Because an electrocardiograph records only a few moments of your heart's action, it may fail to reveal abnormalities that occur infrequently or episodically, such as an irregular heart rhythm. It may be necessary, if you have had a heart attack or have an irregular heart rhythm, to repeat tracings frequently to observe any changes.

Your physician may want to do an *ambulatory cardiogram*, which means you must carry a small, portable recording device (called a *Holter ambulatory monitor*) that continuously traces your heart's rhythm over an extended period, usually twenty-four hours. This is more likely than an ordinary ECG to reveal an episodic change in heart rhythm that may be the cause of dizziness or fainting spells. Although somewhat less convenient than a standard ECG, this prolonged tracing can give invaluable information as to the cause of unusual symptoms. Sometimes the attacks are so infrequent that it may take more than one tracing before the diagnosis can be made. It may also be repeated to see if treatment is effective.

Some people have chest pain that is not typical of angina pectoris. The standard ECG, which is taken while you are resting, may not reveal any abnormalities, so cardiographic tracings may be taken while you exercise in a carefully controlled situation. This is called an *exercise* or *stress* ECG. The tests involve riding a stationary bicycle or walking at increasing speeds on a moving ramp. You will be hooked to an electrocardiograph, and a technician and physician will supervise the examination and interpret the results.

The only danger of this test is that you may experience an episode of angina pain during the procedure. However, it is certainly safer to have an attack under supervision so that a definite diagnosis can be made than to experience attacks when you are alone. Sometimes this test may be repeated after you have been given treatment for your anginal symptoms.

The results of this test are not completely foolproof. You may have a normal test and still suffer from coronary heart disease. Occasionally, a test appears to substantiate heart disease in a person who is normal. The examination itself is only one part of the total evaluation of heart disease. Your doctor will interpret all the tests together before he makes a diagnosis and decides on treatment.

ELECTROENCEPHALOGRAM (EEG)

The diagnosis of various diseases of the brain can sometimes be difficult. X-rays and scans of the skull, including the CAT scan, can determine if there are any changes in the shape of the brain or if there is pressure on it. However, its function is not determined by these tests.

An *electroencephalogram* (EEG), which measures *brain waves,* can be useful in determining the cause of diseases of the nervous system, as well as to follow the results of treatment. Several small wires are attached to the skull, and while you are at rest or even sleeping, your brain waves are recorded. There is no danger or discomfort from this test.

If there is a disorder of the nerves coming from the spinal cord, it may be necessary to measure the efficiency with which they are working. In *nerve conduction* and *muscle studies* very small needles are placed into small nerves and muscles under the skin and their impulses are recorded. These tests can help determine if a symptom such as weakness of a limb is the result of an abnormality of the nerves, rather than from the muscles themselves. There is no danger and minimal discomfort in these tests.

PART TWO

The No-Age-Limit Medical Adviser

CHAPTER 7

Common Complaints

Older people frequently go to their doctor with more than one complaint. Perhaps numerous symptoms began simultaneously or the illness developed in a step-wise fashion: You may have more than one problem, and the symptoms of the first illness may be added to those of a new one. Often, people fail to see the relationship between different symptoms.

As you grow older, illnesses may not be as apparent as during your younger years. If complaints are vague, they may not be associated easily with specific diseases. Therefore, it will help your physician make a diagnosis if you can give him a careful description of your ailment. The symptoms should be outlined and described clearly and, whenever possible, they should be documented as to their frequency and duration.

The emphasis in this section will be on the symptoms of common complaints and not on the details of the illnesses responsible for them. You should use this chapter to help understand the possible causes of your complaints and how to describe them accurately to your doctor. (Consult the Table of

Contents or the Index for the pages where the illnesses or disorders responsible for the symptoms are discussed in detail.)

The first step in good medical care depends on the sympathy and ability of your physician, combined with the cooperation and clarity that you can bring to your medical interview. There is no substitute for these qualities. Although we know that certain bodily processes change with age, all abnormal symptoms are the result of disorders or illnesses and are not caused by age alone. Therefore, you should always receive an adequate explanation of your complaints, based on a full evaluation of your physical and emotional health. And it must always take into account any medications that you are taking for other medical problems. (See Chapter 1 for a complete discussion of what you should do before going to the doctor and what information you should present to him during your visit.)

WEAKNESS

Getting older should not cause you to lose your vigor. However, *weakness* is one of the most common symptoms that affects older individuals. It is so nonspecific that physicians and families often discount the complaint as being the consequence of age. In many cases the difficulty arises because you have trouble explaining exactly what you *mean* by weakness. If the feeling is vague, your physician will need your help to unravel the seemingly puzzling cause. When you complain of weakness, try to be exact. Many symptoms are inadvertently called weakness, but if they are described more accurately—for example, shortness of breath, dizziness, or pain in the legs—your physician can more easily determine the cause.

Loss of muscle strength is one of the frequent causes of the complaint of weakness. In this situation you can usually describe the weariness as being specifically in your lower or upper limbs. Usually the debility comes on after a certain amount of physical activity. You may recognize it when you compare it to previous levels of exertion that you could do comfortably. Now, the same amount of exercise might lead to discomfort or fatigue. You may complain that you cannot lift your legs or arms, as when climbing stairs, putting something on a shelf, or getting out of a chair.

Sometimes all the limbs are affected; at other times only an arm, hand, or leg may be disabled. The symptom may vary throughout the day or be constant. It may have gotten worse over weeks or months, or it may have remained the same. This type of weakness is often the result of disorders of the nervous system or the muscles themselves.

Quite often you may complain of feeling weak when, in fact, you are experiencing *shortness of breath*. Usually the symptom has developed gradually. You may no longer be able to undertake a certain activity, such as walking or running, without feeling "winded." You may feel a need to "breathe more," or you may experience a "lack of air."

When you describe your infirmity, try to explain what your breathing is like at the end of a period of exertion. If you are a homemaker, for example, do you have to stop vacuuming between rooms because you are panting? Do you notice that after you climb only a few stairs you are huffing and puffing and must stop on the landing for a few moments? Have you found that you cannot keep up with your grandchildren on the playground because you must catch your breath? Breathlessness leading to fatigue is usually the result of disorders of the lungs or heart, and not to the effects of age.

Certain types of *pain* are often incorrectly called weakness by older people, particularly if the discomfort has been around for a long time. This is also the case if the pain is a nagging, nonspecific aching or heavy quality rather than sudden and sharp. For example, you may find that you do not have the energy to carry your groceries home from the supermarket. You may have to stop for a few moments because you feel a heaviness in your chest or maybe only in your arm. If you put your bundles down and shake your arm a few times, you may find that you can carry your packages the rest of the way. You may describe this sensation as weakness, when, in fact, the discomfort may be the pain of *angina pectoris.*

Disease of the blood vessels that impairs the circulation to the legs or some types of arthritis and rheumatism can cause pain that may be mistakenly called weakness. You may not be able to walk because your legs feel heavy or uncomfortable which you may interpret as weakness.

Dizziness, attacks of giddiness, and spells of lightheadedness are frequently erroneously described as weakness. You may develop a fear of falling because of these episodes, and they may interfere with your independence. If they occur frequently, you may feel too weak to go out on your own. This symptom is nonspecific, especially in elderly people. It has many causes, including heart disorders and blood pressure control. In most instances, when properly defined, it can be treated effectively.

One of the most important and frequently overlooked factors leading to weakness is a psychological or emotional disturbance. For example, a lack of motivation may be described as weakness. If you find that your life has become empty because there is little that interests you, you may say that you are "weak," rather than express your disappointment in what life seems to be offering. If you know that something cannot be achieved, you may cease to desire it altogether.

One older immigrant woman moved to a city where her children and grandchildren lived, leaving behind her network of friends and social involvements. However, she had not realized before the move that her children had their own interests and activities and could spend relatively little time with her. She was sent to me for an evaluation of her complaint of weakness. She had not been eating well because she was living alone and had developed a mild degree of anemia. After this was corrected, although she said she felt better, she continued to complain of being fatigued. Her family admitted that she "just wasn't doing anything."

After a discussion with her about her expectations and activities, it became clear that she had put all of her hopes for activity into her family. She was directed to a number of senior-citizen centers, where she was able to get involved again in activities that interested and stimulated her. The "weakness" gradually disappeared as her social involvement increased.

Another important psychological cause of fatigue and lack of energy is *depression*. This important and frequently overlooked disorder can cause serious problems, and the diagnosis is often disregarded because the symptoms are different from those in younger people. You may lose your interest in outside activities and say that you are "tired" and would rather stay home and "rest." Your family may encourage you to join in, and this may only aggravate your feelings. The recognition of depression as a cause of fatigue and weakness is of utmost importance. Misdiagnosis can lead to inappropriate treatment and even to decisions that may affect your living arrangements.

PAIN

Although the experience and appreciation of pain is very complex, we have recently begun to understand more about the brain's ability to feel pain and how medications to treat pain work. For discomfort to be experienced, there must be some abnormal stimulus to a part of the body. The outside as well as the inside of the body is generously supplied with nerves that can become irritated. If there is a trigger, such as pressure, squeezing, excess heat or cold, or cutting or impairment of oxygen supply, the nerves will send impulses to the brain.

We usually experience pain at a conscious level, although certain reflexes react to pain even before we are aware of it. When you accidentally put your hand on a hot stove, you will remove it quickly a few seconds before you actually realize just how much you have burned yourself. This is part of a natural protective mechanism that works faster than our conscious awareness of pain. When the brain receives a pain stimulus, it interprets and modifies it. We all know some people who appear to bear pain more stoically than others. Personality factors allow some people to withstand greater amounts of discomfort.

Analgesics can modify or dispel pain. A local anesthetic applied to the skin after a burn or injected into the gums before dental work prevents the nerves from passing the painful stimuli to the brain. If you suffer from pain because of a swollen, inflamed, arthritic joint, the removal of fluid and injection of a medication like cortisone, which decreases inflammation, may relieve your discomfort.

Some types of pain are more difficult to bear than others. In many instances the fear of pain or the recollection of a previous painful experience can be frightening. Some medications affect the brain in order to relieve pain. There are naturally occurring substances called *endorphins* that exist in the brain and modify the appreciation of pain. Some of the drugs used to treat severe pain, such as morphine, probably work partially by stimulating the body's own endorphins to modify pain. There is a great deal more to learn about pain. The use of *acupuncture* and *hypnosis* to relieve pain have been successful in some people. How they work is unclear. More research is necessary to discover how pain is caused and how it can best be relieved in each individual.

Most of us appreciate that pain is often a symptom of an injury or an illness. It is one of the first questions asked at every medical interview. Because we have all experienced various types of pain during our lives, it is common for people to treat certain types of discomfort by themselves without going to a doctor. As people grow older, the interpretation of pain may alter. It may be more subtle and less characteristic than in younger people. Because of this, you may not seek medical attention as quickly or as intently as you should. The severity or implication of pain may not be appreciated by you, your family, or your physician, and this could lead to a delay in diagnosis and treatment.

One usually thinks of pain as being of recent onset *(acute)* or long-standing *(chronic)*. It is acute pain that usually brings patients for urgent medical attention because it is more frightening and sinister than pain that has started gradually or has been going on for a long time.

The appreciation of pain is variable. Some older people appear to react more to a given amount of pain than others. It is therefore difficult for someone else, professional or non-professional, to appreciate the pain that you describe. This, however, should not interfere with proper medical attention. Physicians are aware of the patterns of pain that occur with illness without necessarily having personally experienced it themselves. I have often heard patients exclaim to me while I was trying to diagnose the cause of their pain, "You can't understand what I am feeling unless you have had it yourself." This is not so, and it does not interfere with the physician's ability to diagnose its cause or treat it effectively.

Acute pain may arise from any part of the body, usually because of a rapid change of function. Some examples of acute pain are those following an injury resulting in bruised muscles, fractured bones, damage to the heart, increased pressure within the skull, and irritation of nerves in the lungs or bowel. Severe discomfort may be caused by many illnesses, including inflammation or loss of blood supply. If you experience an attack of pain that you have never felt before, and if it lasts for more than a few moments and is not easily explainable by a simple event, seek medical advice as soon as possible.

Chronic pain may cause greater disability than acute pain because the latter leads to immediate medical advice and treatment. Long-standing pain can result from illnesses that are partially irreversible. Their progress may be insidious and gradual, or perhaps the pain previously responded to various analgesics. One problem with chronic pain is that your repeated complaints about it may fall on deaf ears. As your sufferings go unheeded, you may acquiesce and simply change pain pills without seeking proper treatment.

The main types of chronic pain include those from various forms of arthritis and rheumatism, long-standing abnormalities of the stomach and bowel, some types of heart disease, and malignant tumors. Pain from the stomach and bowel (gastrointestinal system) or heart and blood vessels (cardiovascular system) can be treated by special medications. If you suffer from the chest pain of angina pectoris, you may get relief by decreasing your activity or taking a nitroglycerin tablet when the pain occurs. Or your physician might tell you to take the nitroglycerin tablet before activity that produces the pain in an attempt to prevent it. He may also recommend weight loss as a measure to decrease the heart's work, and this can also relieve the pain.

The same rule applies to the treatment of chronic pain from arthritis and rheumatism. These conditions often respond better to repeated doses of antiinflammatory or analgesic medications taken even when there is no pain. This may be more effective than waiting for the pain to occur. You should never treat undiagnosed pain on your own. Any persistent pain or discomfort, especially if it is not easily relieved by simple analgesics, should be evaluated by a physician. I have seen patients take aspirin for abdominal discomfort that was the result of a stomach ulcer. The pain was not relieved and the aspirin may even have aggravated the ulcer.

FEVER

The body's temperature is controlled very carefully, and becoming excessively cold or warm can cause damage. We usually associate fever with illness, but usually the illness causing the raised temperature is short-lived and improves with or without medication. In the older individual especially, an elevated temperature may have a number of causes, but it is usually the result of an infection, as is the case in people of all ages. Infections from bacteria and viruses almost invariably cause fever.

In some older people, however, there is an abnormality in the temperature-regulating mechanism. This may lead to an excessive rise of temperature with an infection, or it can occur if you have spent too much time in the sun or in an extremely warm environment. The opposite also occurs. A severe infection may be present without causing an elevation in your temperature.

Whenever you have a fever from an infection, there are usually other symptoms that point to the source of the illness. Bacterial infections of the urinary tract usually cause burning when you pass urine and an urgency to urinate frequently. A lung infection often leads to coughing and the production of phlegm. We usually recognize the muscle aches and pains of a cold or influenza, and the fever usually subsides by itself within a few days. The fever caused by bacterial infections usually decreases after treatment with antibiotics has begun to be effective.

Some unusual illnesses in older people can cause fever that is not the result of infections. These ailments often lead to the greatest confusion in diagnosis and treatment. Unlike most infectious causes of temperature elevation, despite treatment with a few days of aspirin or an antibiotic, the elevated temperature does not return to normal. Sometimes the temperature goes up and down, either daily or weekly. At times it may even stay up for a week or two and then fall to normal for a few weeks and then go up again.

Various types of inflammation and certain tumors, especially of the blood or lymph glands, can cause fever. The temperature can also be elevated during unusual infections, such as bacterial endocarditis or tuberculosis. In these circumstances the temperature will not decrease with the usual fever-lowering medications such as aspirin, or if it does, it will return soon after. Antibiotics may not lower the temperature, or will do so only temporarily, and the fever may return again after the medication is stopped.

An illness accompanied by fever should be carefully evaluated. Most of us recognize such simple causes of temperature elevation as a cold or influenza. If you have a fever that does not fall within a few days, or if it returns time after time, whether or not you have taken medications such as antibiotics, you should have a full examination and explanation from your physician. It is very dangerous for you to treat yourself with antibiotics repeatedly, especially if after a course of treatment your fever returns.

INSOMNIA

Sleep is a very important activity, and every day we learn more and more about the body's need for sleep and its many positive physical and emotional effects. Older people often feel that they are not getting enough sleep, or they become frustrated and anxious that sleep does not come easily. As a consequence, unfortunately, sleeping medications account for one of the most frequently prescribed drugs in the elderly.

As we age, less sleep may be required for the mind and body to work properly. For most individuals a sleep pattern is established early in life, and this usually continues into the later years. You may be used to going to bed at a certain hour, perhaps with your spouse or after a favorite television program. Then you sleep until morning. Some of your sleep requirements may be met by afternoon naps, which you may not think of as "sleep."

Sleeping medications give only a temporary improvement in sleep patterns. Most medications work when first taken, but gradually their effect wears off. This may lead you to take larger doses and stronger sleeping pills. Your physician may prescribe tranquilizers instead of sleeping pills in the hope of calming you into sleep. Tolerance to these drugs also diminishes and they lose their soporific effect. They often accumulate in the body and may lead to mental confusion, memory impairment, and dizziness.

If you are taking sleeping pills, you should try to discontinue them. Patterns of sleep can be relearned. You could try going to sleep much later than you usually do. A warm drink such as milk may be helpful in soothing your mind and body. Reading a book or listening to music can also have a calming effect. If sleep does not come easily, get out of bed and read, knit, or do something else, rather than lie in bed anxiously waiting to fall asleep.

You may have difficulty sleeping because of a medical problem. Arthritic pain, the need to run to the bathroom frequently, or shortness of breath can interfere with your sleep. But taking a sleeping pill will not help, and it may even aggravate some of your other symptoms. Sleep disturbance is a common symptom in people who suffer from depression. The problem may be one of falling asleep or of sleeping fitfully and waking up early in the morning. Tranquilizers and sleeping pills usually make the depression worse.

When your sleep pattern has changed suddenly, your physician should pursue the cause. You should avoid taking a sleeping pill as a solution. Most people can enjoy a restful sleep without the use of tranquilizers and sleeping pills.

WEIGHT GAIN

Once we reach adulthood, we usually maintain a fairly steady weight. Weight can go up during the middle years, especially if your exercise and physical activity is minimal. Beyond middle age your weight may drop slightly because the size of your skeleton and the bulk of your muscles gradually decreases. In Western countries excess weight is a common problem, and it may become exaggerated with age. But it is not normal or healthy.

The most common cause of weight gain is a decrease in activity compared to the number of calories eaten. Since eating habits rarely change, and as the inclination to exercise often decreases with age, many older people tend to gain weight.

This may be exaggerated by economic factors, which force an increased reliance on sugars, starches (carbohydrates), and fats when good sources of protein become prohibitively expensive. Besides decreasing your energy level, excess weight has serious consequences on your ability to function well: It increases the work of the heart, exaggerates the symptoms of arthritic conditions and back pain, increases the risks in surgery, and makes diabetes mellitus more difficult to control.

The most effective way to deal with weight gain is to maintain a reasonable degree of activity and carefully limit your food intake. The best way to assure adequate physical activity is to prepare in advance for your senior years by developing good exercise habits. Even if you have never been used to physical exertion, it is never too late to start on a program of gradually increasing exercise. This will also improve your sense of well-being.

If you are overweight, you should try to reduce, even though it is difficult to change eating patterns that were developed over many years. Group sessions such as those given by senior-citizen organizations, weight-reduction associations, or by dietitians and physicians may be helpful in guiding your eating habits. It is important to avoid fats (especially animal fats), sugars, and starches and substitute protein and high-fiber vegetables, which have low caloric value.

Far too often an older person becomes aware of the disability resulting from obesity only after having suffered from a serious illness or surgery. It should not be necessary to learn the hard way that being overweight can endanger your health and even your life.

Some causes of weight gain may be the result of illnesses rather than an imbalance between food intake and physical activity. Whenever your pattern of weight changes unexpectedly or if you have other symptoms in addition to weight gain, consult your physician.

Elderly persons with heart disease may gain weight because water tends to accumulate throughout the body. You may become aware of swelling of your legs and abdomen, which may vary throughout the day, with a tendency to worsen in the evening and improve after a night's sleep. You may feel short of breath or experience other heart symptoms. Because the weight gain can be gradual, the connection between heart disease and fluid accumulation may be overlooked.

People with an underactive thyroid gland (hypothyroidism) may also experience weight gain. This illness may be very gradual in its onset. You may or may not be aware of a generalized slowing of your physical and mental condition, or you experience weight gain despite a limited food intake.

Heart disease, an underactive thyroid gland, and other causes of fluid retention should be looked for and proper treatment sought whenever there is unexpected weight gain. This usually results in a loss of the excess weight.

WEIGHT LOSS

With the great emphasis on weight control, one would assume that weight loss is a welcome relief from the tendency toward obesity that plagues many older individuals. Your body will usually maintain its weight so long as there is no major change in food intake or degree of physical activity. If you consciously want to lose weight, you will no doubt change your eating habits or activities. The weight loss is not only expected, but anticipated and welcomed.

But sometimes you might begin to lose weight despite maintaining a steady degree of physical activity and a well-balanced diet. When this happens, weight loss may be the first sign of an illness that may present no other symptoms, especially in the early stages. The point at which you might begin to notice your weight loss depends on your lifestyle. If you live in an institution, weight loss may be noticed early if the staff weighs you regularly. If you live at home and do not weigh yourself periodically, the first sign may be that your clothes are loose. Neighbors, friends, or relatives may remark that you look thinner. Or your physician may notice your loss of weight since your previous visit.

If you are certain that you have not changed your food intake or physical activity, you should look for other symptoms that may be causing the weight loss. Medical advice should be sought.

A number of illnesses can lead to a loss of weight despite a good appetite and a normal diet. An overactive thyroid gland (hyperthyroidism) in the older person may show itself as weight loss without the symptoms that are usually found in younger people. You may experience heart palpitations and emotional irritability or perhaps some loosening of the bowel movement. Frequently, however, weight loss is the only symptom.

Long-standing (chronic) infections, such as tuberculosis and bacterial endocarditis (heart infections), can also lead to weight loss. There is usually fever and a general feeling of debilitation, as well as a loss of appetite.

If you are aware of what is often called *occult malignancy* (hidden cancer), also a cause of weight loss, you may become frightened and postpone medical advice. However, many other hidden noncancerous conditions can lead to the same symptoms. Even a cancer that shows itself as weight loss might be treatable. It is more likely to respond to therapy if discovered early than if allowed to progress until other symptoms appear. Never let your fears keep you from getting proper advice.

If you take *digoxin* and *diuretics* (water pills) for heart failure, you may lose weight. This is, in fact, excess fluid. You usually can associate your "dry weight" (after fluid is lost) with the improvement in heart symptoms and the disappearance of the swelling in your legs and abdomen.

Occasionally an older person develops diabetes mellitus and experiences weight loss with an increase in appetite and in the amount of urine passed. However, more commonly in the older person, diabetes mellitus is accompanied by obesity.

Malabsorption, in which food is not absorbed properly, may be the result of some problem within the bowel itself or within the pancreas, which manufactures enzymes (digestive helpers). Sometimes the pancreas does not produce enough enzymes, and the food is poorly digested in the intestine and therefore poorly absorbed. You may or may not have diarrhea. The inability to absorb nutrients leads to a gradual loss of weight just the same as if you stopped eating.

LOSS OF APPETITE

Losing your appetite can be very discouraging, and it is a common complaint of older people. You may ask your doctor or pharmacist for a "tonic" to improve your appetite, and you may get a mixture of vitamins and alcohol, which acts for a short period only as a placebo.

A decreased or lost appetite can be caused by various physical and psychological illnesses or be a side effect of medication. Some drugs affect the appetite more than others. *Digoxin,* used for heart diseases, can accumulate in your body and lead to *digitalis toxicity,* which often results in a loss of appetite. Other medications that can lead to appetite loss include antibiotics, especially tetracycline and erythromycin, drugs used to treat Parkinson's disease, heart palpitations (irregular heart rhythms), or abnormal emotional states.

In addition to drugs many illnesses can lead to a loss of appetite, including those that affect the stomach, bowel, liver, and pancreas. Diseased kidneys may cause a gradual loss of appetite, as may an underactive or overactive thyroid gland and metabolic disturbances affecting the body's control of calcium.

A major cause of appetite loss is depression. This illness may not be immediately recognized by you, your family, or your physician because the symptoms are often different from those in the younger person. If you think you are suffering from depression, consult your physician, who can prescribe antidepressant therapy.

You should always be on the lookout for social situations that interfere with your desire to eat. If you live alone, you may lose interest in preparing food or you may not want to eat because you have no one to share a meal with. This is similar to depression, but it can be treated by finding friends or neighbors to eat with.

Although as you get older your needs for food may decrease, you should not confuse this with appetite loss. If your weight remains steady, there is usually little to worry about. When loss of appetite is severe, it usually causes weight loss, which should be evaluated by a physician.

One 93-year-old lady caused great concern in her daughters because she ate very little according to their standards. They said she only nibbled at her food, whereas she claimed that she ate all that she needed. She remarked, "At 93 you don't need much food." A comparison of weights taken at my office showed that she was the exact weight two years previously. Clearly she knew what she was talking about.

HEARTBURN

There are many terms to describe heartburn, a very common complaint. It is a sensation of burning or bitterness in the middle of the chest and the back of the throat. In some countries it is known as *water-brash* or *acid indigestion*, whereas we refer to it as heartburn.

Acid is normally produced by the stomach and is used in the digestion of food. The connection between the esophagus and stomach is guarded by a valve (sphincter) that prevents acid from going out of the stomach into the esophagus and up into the throat or mouth. When the valve does not work properly, some excess acid may enter the esophagus, causing heartburn. Some older individuals produce an increased amount of acid. They often suffer from *acid-peptic disease*, which may cause stomach or duodenal ulcers or aggravate a *hiatus hernia.* In the latter, a part of the stomach goes above the diaphragm (the breathing muscle that separates the chest from the abdomen), and prevents the valve from keeping the acid in the stomach.

There are a number of ways to treat heartburn. In some people it is aggravated by various foods or stimulants, such as alcohol, caffeine, and cigarettes. You may learn that certain foods intensify your heartburn and other foods relieve it. Milk products and other bland foods often improve the symptoms.

If you suffer heartburn from a hiatus hernia, you know that it is aggravated by overeating, lying down, bending over, or wearing excessively tight clothing or girdles. You may have noticed that when you are overweight the symptoms of heartburn are worse and when you lose weight there is relief.

In most instances people suffer from heartburn only occasionally. You usually can treat yourself with a dose of a liquid or tablet antacid, a glass of milk, or by avoiding foods that make your symptoms worse. For some, heartburn may be intolerable. It can interfere with the enjoyment of food, sleep, and the activities of daily life. If this is so, you should find out if the symptoms are related to ulcer disease or to a *symptomatic* hiatus hernia. Tests and X-rays of the esophagus and stomach are usually done to determine the cause. You may be X-rayed with your head down to show that the stomach acid refluxes (passes through the sphincter) and goes from the stomach into the esophagus.

Sometimes your physician will use a *gastroscope* to look into the stomach to see whether he can prove that stomach acid is backing up into the esophagus. In severe cases he may prescribe frequent doses of liquid antacids. There are also new medications to decrease the acid production by the stomach (*cimetidine*) or to improve the closure of the valve that separates the stomach from the esophagus (*metoclopramide*). These drugs often improve the symptoms, and they can be used alone or with antacids.

Rarely does an older person with severe heartburn from a hiatus hernia require surgery for the relief of symptoms.

Surgery is usually necessary only if the medications are not effective or you become severely disabled and no longer enjoy food or routine activities.

INDIGESTION

Indigestion means different things to different people. To many, it is just another word to describe heartburn. To others, it is used to describe any pain or discomfort that occurs in the abdomen around mealtime. Although abdominal pain can occur before eating, most people experience indigestion after a meal. Whether you experience it immediately after a meal or some time after depends on the cause.

There are numerous reasons for indigestion other than heartburn. Pain from ulcer disease, which can be severe, usually occurs in the mid-part of the upper abdomen and perhaps goes toward the back. A change in diet or the use of antacid medications usually helps.

If you have disease of the gallbladder and biliary tree (the connections from the gallbladder to the liver and intestine), you may be sensitive to certain types of food, particularly fried and fatty foods. The discomfort occurs in the upper right side of the abdomen after you have eaten an excessively fatty meal.

Some older people have a poor blood supply to their intestines and may have discomfort following meals. This is similar to angina pectoris, where the blood supply to the heart is not adequate for the demands of excess physical activity. This problem is often confused with other symptoms of indigestion or abdominal pain and may be difficult to diagnose.

Indigestion often describes the various nonspecific feelings, such as bloating, fullness, or heaviness, that sometimes occur following a meal. Some older people tend to swallow air, which also causes these symptoms. Occasionally, a blockage of the large bowel can cause abdominal bloating following meals. Usually you will be aware of a change in bowel habit. Some individuals with *lactose intolerance* experience bloating, abdominal cramps, and loose bowel movements when they eat milk products. Very often no cause is found other than the psychological stresses that you may experience as you grow older. Occasionally, the discomfort of angina pectoris is confused with indigestion.

To find the cause of indigestion, many tests may be required if the symptoms have not been relieved by simple measures. In most instances an investigation of the gastrointestinal tract is necessary. The tests may include *gallbladder X-rays* (oral cholecystogram and intravenous cholangiogram) and an *upper G.I. series (barium swallow), sigmoidoscopy,* and *barium enema.* Treatment may include changes in diet or the use of antacids or the newer medications such as cimetidine or metoclopramide.

Surgery for gallbladder disease is recommended if there has been an infection of the gallbladder or an attack of gallstones that has caused a severe pain or blockage to the flow of bile. If an X-ray shows that you have gallstones, this does not necessarily mean that they are causing your symptoms, and this will be determined before surgery is considered.

CONSTIPATION

Older people often claim that they are constipated. It is difficult to define what is "normal" when it comes to bowel habits. You were brought up at a time when ideas about bowel movements led to some unnatural and unhealthy practices, such as the use of cathartics (purges) and laxatives. Many people grew up with the idea that a frequent "cleaning out" was essential for health. This was often combined with a decreasing amount of fiber (roughage) in the diet.

As the years of frequent laxative use pass, your bowel may become insensitive to the various types. It is common to enter a cycle in which you become more and more dependent on increasingly stronger laxatives. The bowel movement seems to be less likely to result in a feeling of relief or comfort. Some people spend a great deal of time and a good deal of their visits to the doctor describing their bowel problems. There is an endless search for that magic formula for a good daily bowel movement and freedom from constipation. However, a bowel movement does not have to occur every day for you to be healthy. Some normal older people have a bowel movement only every two or three days. What is important is that when you do have a bowel movement, it is not excessively hard and does not cause discomfort.

It is important to distinguish between constipation as a result of a *change in bowel habit* and constipation that has existed for many years, or *chronic constipation*. The former may be an early sign of blockage of the intestine, sometimes from an inflammation or a tumor. If you have a change in bowel habits, you should consult your physician as soon as possible. If you suffer from long-standing and progressive constipation, you should be examined for an underactive thyroid gland (hypothyroidism). Sometimes local causes, such as hemorrhoids or fissures (sores in the anus), exaggerate a tendency toward constipation.

If your physician finds that your constipation is caused by poor bowel habits, an attempt should be made at retraining the bowel. You should try to discontinue the use of laxatives, which excessively stimulate the bowel, and replace them with safer substances, such as *psyllium mucilloid* or *lactulose*. You should make sure that your diet contains sufficient fiber in the form of bran, whole-wheat and other whole-grain breads and cereals, raw and cooked vegetables, and fruits, as well as an adequate intake of fluids. This gives the lower intestine enough bulk to stimulate a normal bowel movement. The ultimate goal is to have a bowel movement of sufficient frequency so that it is well formed, not excessively hard, and easy to expel. But it does not have to be a daily occurrence.

A change in behavior may also be helpful. You should try to

have a bowel movement following meals and try not to hurry. It is advisable to avoid enemas. However, while you wean yourself from laxatives, if a normal pattern does not become quickly established, an occasional enema is preferable to a strong laxative. Increasing your physical activity is also beneficial in breaking the constipation cycle.

DIARRHEA

Whereas most people experience one or two bowel movements daily, others may have one only every few days. These patterns are all normal according to each individual. The term *diarrhea* is usually reserved for bowel movements that are excessively frequent and tend to be watery and poorly controlled. The onset may be sudden or gradual, and the degree of looseness may vary from time to time.

Diarrhea should be considered abnormal when it is different from your usual bowel movement pattern. Even though it may come as a relief after many years of constipation, the experience of new diarrhea should be taken seriously. If it continues for more than a short period or if it returns frequently, medical advice should be sought. Any degree of diarrhea that begins to interfere with the normal activities of your life or shows mucus or blood must be checked immediately.

One of the common causes of diarrhea is infection. Various viruses ("stomach flu") and bacteria can infect your bowel and cause diarrhea. Usually you will have other evidence of infection, such as fever and abdominal pain. The diarrhea is usually short-lived and does not recur.

An older person also may suffer from inflammatory bowel disease, even though it is more common in younger people. The diarrhea is often combined with mucus and blood, and you may have other symptoms as well, such as fever. It usually persists, unlike infectious diarrhea, until properly diagnosed and treated.

Malabsorption may appear initially as loose bowel movements. It may take some time before you become aware of weight loss, which is usually associated with poor absorption and digestion of food.

If you have traveled a great deal or lived under unhygienic conditions, you may suffer from *parasites,* which can cause diarrhea. The diarrhea often contains red blood.

An often overlooked cause of diarrhea in older individuals is *lactose intolerance,* the result of a lack of the lactase enzyme that normally breaks up lactose, the sugar found in milk. Therefore, milk products are not properly digested and the sugar is fermented by the bacteria in the intestine. The symptoms include bloating, gas, abdominal cramps, and frequent loose bowel movements. If you are observant, you may see that your symptoms often follow meals in which milk products are eaten. Remember, although you avoid milk, yogurt, and cheese, many packaged foods, including bread, contain milk.

Some people with lactose intolerance may spontaneously improve periodically and may be able to tolerate small amounts of milk products. However, if you suffer from a bout of stomach flu, you may no longer be able to endure milk products and once again develop bowel symptoms.

If you overuse and abuse laxatives, you may develop diarrhea that alternates with constipation and take a further dose of laxative to relieve the constipation. You may then experience diarrhea that, in fact, is a result of excess laxative use. This is very common in older people. You should avoid laxatives and seek advice from your physician.

With a bowel obstruction, sometimes the only material that can pass through the blockage is liquid stool, which appears as diarrhea. Medication may relieve it, but this only exaggerates the obstruction and is dangerous. Diarrhea that alternates with constipation should be investigated thoroughly.

Because many possible reasons for diarrhea exist, there is no single effective treatment. The most important step is to find the underlying cause, and unless it is clearly the result of a temporary problem such as flu, which can be expected to improve within a few days, *diarrhea should not be treated with constipating agents.*

The short-term therapy consists of decreasing food intake and eating a primarily liquid diet. Soups, juices, and tea are recommended during the treatment of the kind of diarrhea that often occurs with bowel infections. If you are in the habit of taking laxatives, you should consult your physician about stopping them. If the diarrhea continues despite discontinuing laxatives, your physician should investigate the cause. This should be done without delay if the diarrhea persists.

INTESTINAL GAS

Intestinal gas includes a number of problems, such as burping, belching, swelling and bloating of the abdomen, and an increase in the passage of "wind" (flatus). These symptoms can be so disturbing that some individuals change their social life in order to avoid the embarrassment that comes with "too much gas."

There are two ways in which gas can enter the digestive system. The most common way is by swallowing air. This occurs unconsciously during eating and drinking and is normal for everyone. Some people, however, swallow too much air, especially when anxious or under stress.

It is common for some older people to swallow air and then immediately burp or belch to relieve certain kinds of abdominal discomfort. People with acid indigestion often develop this habit, and they may even drink carbonated beverages such as soda water to increase the amount of air in their belch.

The other source of intestinal gas is from the fermentation and digestion of food by bacteria that normally inhabit the large intestine. These bacteria break down nutrients, and one of the byproducts is intestinal gas. Everyone produces some gas normally, and for the most part this is passed without problem, either during a bowel movement or discreetly throughout the day.

Some people seem to be plagued by abdominal swelling and bloating as well as pain. In fact, studies have shown that the amount of gas in the intestine is about the same in all individuals. It appears that some people become more sensitive to normal amounts of gas, and when the bowel is stretched by the gas, it becomes uncomfortable and results in a bloating sensation.

Since almost all gas entering the esophagus and stomach comes from what you swallow, the most important step in decreasing burping and belching is to learn how to swallow less air. You can begin by avoiding carbonated beverages, which contain excess amounts of gas. Eat meals slowly, and never gulp liquids. Avoid chewing gum and smoking, which can lead to increased amounts of swallowed air. If you suffer from acid indigestion, relieve it with antacids.

The passing of malodorous wind is very disquieting to some people. All of us have to pass a certain amount of flatus as part of our normal bodily functions. If, however, you tend to swallow air, the amount of flatus will increase. In addition, certain foods will produce excessive amounts of gas and increase the undesirable odor. Therefore, after your physician has determined that no illnesses are affecting your bowel, a change of diet is often helpful.

You should try to eat smaller meals more frequently rather than one or two large meals a day. If you take liquids with your meals, they should be in smaller amounts, and you should drink them slowly rather than using them to "wash down" the food. You should also try to eat slowly. If you have a *lactose intolerance*, a decrease in milk products will be helpful.

You should avoid chewing gum or sucking candies, and you should stop smoking. Some foods, such as beans, nuts, cauliflower, cabbage, broccoli, radishes, turnips, apples, and other raw fruits and vegetables, may lead to an increase in gas. However, rather than discontinuing these foods simultaneously, it might be necessary only to decrease or omit a few of them. Try one at a time and see the result. Many of these foods also supply important amounts of fiber, vitamins, and minerals, and stopping them altogether could lead to serious nutritional problems.

Medications such as antacids decrease the amount of gas. *Simethicone*, which is often combined with antacids, allows swallowed air to be belched, rather than having it pass through the intestine and leave the body as flatus. You should avoid laxatives because some increase gas. No medication, however, can completely cure excess flatus.

Although many medications, one being *chlorophyllin*, have been used to decrease the objectionable odor that is associated with excess flatus, none has proven to be successful in all people. Some people benefit from certain medications if changes in their diet and eating habits have not been beneficial. Chlorophyllin can be taken if you feel that the odor of your flatus and stool is so objectionable that it is interfering with your emotional and social life. Although chlorophyllin is not readily available, your physician can arrange to have your pharmacist order it for you. It will make your stool green, but it does not appear to have any other negative effects.

CHEST PAIN

Chest pain is one of the most frightening symptoms that affects individuals of all ages. In an older person the degree of pain may be less vivid than in a younger person and therefore may go unnoticed. Chest pain is either *acute* (sudden) or *chronic* (long-standing). Acute chest pain has many causes, including illnesses affecting the heart, lungs, and the muscles and bones of the chest and spine. The type of pain often tells the physician the underlying cause.

A common cause of acute chest pain is a heart attack (*myocardial infarction, coronary thrombosis*). Typically, but not

167

necessarily, the pain starts suddenly and is felt behind the breastbone. It is characterized by a pressing or heavy feeling that sometimes goes to the back or to the shoulder and wrist. Occasionally, it is felt in the neck and jaw. You may experience a pain in the lower chest and think it your stomach and mistake it for indigestion. I have seen many older people postpone a visit to their physician because they assumed they were suffering from indigestion when, in fact, they had experienced a heart attack.

Often the pain of a heart attack is less typical in the elderly. One woman came to my office complaining of indigestion, a problem she had had for many years. While she was waiting, the nurse noticed that she was burping frequently, and seemed to be uncomfortable. Based on this, an electrocardiogram was done before I saw her. The tracing showed that she had suffered a myocardial infarction. At no time had she complained of the chest pain that usually accompanies a heart attack.

Other causes for the sudden onset of chest pain are a *pneumothorax* (collapse of a lung), *pulmonary embolism* (blood clot to the lung), or an acute lung infection *(pneumonia)*. Usually, symptoms such as shortness of breath, cough, phlegm, or fever indicate a lung problem. Acute chest pain can also result from spontaneous fractures of the spine and ribs. Older people have a tendency to experience spontaneous fractures of their spine. Sometimes this causes pain in the chest, rather than in the back, because nerves are pinched as they leave the spine and wrap around the chest.

An elderly lady I saw was urgently admitted to the hospital because she had acute pain in her lower chest and upper abdomen. She could not find a comfortable way to lie in bed. An immediate electrocardiogram failed to show evidence of a heart attack to account for her pain. Nitroglycerin did not make the pain go away. X-rays of her spine showed that she had fractured three vertebrae (spinal bones), which probably pressed on the nerves going to the front of her chest. Treatment with painkillers (analgesics) and heat to her back relieved her pain, which eventually subsided on its own.

Chronic chest pain occurs for the same reasons as acute pain. It can come from muscle and bone disorders, such as arthritis, that affect the spine and ribs, or occasionally from bone tumors affecting the spine or ribs. But the most common cause of chronic chest pain is *angina pectoris*, and it occurs when physical activity or emotional stress strains the heart. The pressing or heavy pain in the chest disappears when the exertion or stress is stopped. Your physician can demonstrate the relationship between the pain and an increased demand on the heart by emotional stress and physical activity, or by a common trigger of anginal pain, walking into a cold wind.

A common imitator of angina pectoris in older people is a *hiatus hernia*. Even though the pain typically has a burning quality, which is different from angina pectoris, it can sometimes be indistinguishable from anginal pain. It occurs especially when bending over and at night. Diagnosis often requires X-rays of the stomach and occasionally *gastroscopy*, which shows whether gastric juice is coming from the stomach and irritating the esophagus.

At times, the exact cause of chronic chest pain is difficult to determine, especially if more than one factor is playing a role in its production. Your physician may have to use various drugs in sequence and in combination in order to relieve pain that has multiple and elusive causes.

SHORTNESS OF BREATH

The bloodstream is the body's transportation system for gases. Blood is pumped into the lungs, where it deposits carbon dioxide, a waste product, and receives oxygen. The fine balance and control between the heart and lungs prevents shortness of breath even when you exercise. Shortness of breath (*dyspnea*) that occurs at rest or with little exercise usually means an imbalance between the two. It can be acute or chronic, but in either case it is caused by diseases of the heart or lungs, or both. Occasionally, illnesses such as anemia or excess thyroid hormone (hyperthyroidism) tax the heart so that it must work overtime. The result is shortness of breath.

Sudden breathlessness can occur without warning, and it can be frightening. You may feel that you are choking because you are unable to catch your breath. Depending on the cause, there may also be pain in the chest, cough, heart palpitations, dizziness, lightheadedness, and mental confusion.

One of the common causes of sudden breathlessness is *heart failure.* When it occurs suddenly, it is called acute heart failure, or *pulmonary edema,* and it means that the pumping action of the heart suddenly becomes impaired. Instead of the heart being able to effectively pump the blood that has been brought to it, the blood backs up and collects in the lungs, thereby interfering with the exchange of oxygen and carbon dioxide.

The common causes of acute heart failure are heart attacks (myocardial infarction), a sudden irregularity of the heart rhythm (cardiac arrhythmia), or conditions that suddenly over-tax the heart, such as severe anemia, hyperthyroidism, or a pulmonary embolism. Most often immediate emergency-room care and hospitalization are required. Medications such as diuretics, morphine, and digoxin are used because they drain the fluid from the lungs and improve the efficiency of the heart's pumping action. Tests, including an electrocardiogram, chest X-ray, and blood tests, may be necessary to find the exact cause and best treatment for this condition.

Even though the *pulmonary* (lung) causes of sudden breathlessness can be as dramatic as the *cardiac* (heart) causes, in most cases they are more gradual, even during an acute situation.

A *collapsed lung (pneumothorax)* can also cause sudden breathlessness. In this situation one of the small air sacs in the lung ruptures, and air rushes out of the lung and into the pleural space, between it and the chest wall. The lung loses its air and collapses. Sometimes there is sudden pain with the episode. Chronic bronchitis and emphysema are often responsible for a collapsed lung. Immediate medical attention is required to allow the lung to reexpand.

Other common respiratory causes of sudden breathlessness are infections such as acute bronchitis or pneumonia. You may not know that you have these diseases until your first severe infection. You may have had a recent cold or flu with some cough, phlegm, or fever. Sometimes a rapid progression of symptoms occurs within a few hours and you may become short of breath. The most important clue to a lung infection is coughing and yellowish or green phlegm.

Another condition that causes shortness of breath is a *pulmonary embolism*. A blood clot (thrombus) forms either in the veins of the legs or pelvis and makes its way to the heart and lungs. The clot blocks the blood flow from the heart to the lungs and interferes with breathing. Other symptoms are chest pain and occasionally blood being coughed up. This is a medical emergency that requires hospitalization and rapid treatment with anticoagulants (blood thinners) to prevent further blood clots from forming. Very rarely, emergency surgery is done to remove the blood clot from the lungs.

You are most at risk if you have had surgery or have suffered from a severe illness that has required prolonged bed rest. Operations and fractures, especially when occurring after an accident, put you in the greatest danger. However, there is a good chance for a complete recovery. One spry 93-year-old patient I treated had fractured her hip. She agreed to hip surgery and was doing well until three days after the operation, when she suddenly developed severe pain in her chest and became short of breath. She was diagnosed as having a pulmonary embolus. Despite her age, she withstood the illness very well and made an excellent recovery. Three years later, she is still an active, involved, and very independent woman.

A number of less common events can cause sudden

breathlessness. In some, following an inflammatory illness or viral infection, the lungs accumulate excess scar tissue. For some unknown reason, the body tries to counteract the inflammation and produces a jelly-like material which fills the lungs and interferes with their proper function.

Inhaling a noxious material during a fire or breathing some chemical that may inflame the lung can cause sudden breathlessness. These conditions are usually job-related and rarely occur in older people.

In most cases of sudden breathlessness, hospitalization is required for proper investigation and treatment. First-aid measures by a physician or in an emergency room can be life-saving, such as relieving the air from the chest in a pneumothorax, improving the severe fluid congestion in heart failure, or giving oxygen after removing a person from a smoke-filled room. Most of these conditions respond to treatment, but urgent medical attention improves the chances of recovery.

Unlike the sudden causes of shortness of breath, the *chronic* causes may be gradual and therefore more insidious. It may take many days, weeks, or months before you are aware that you no longer can undertake your normal activities because of shortness of breath.

If you have heart disease, you may discover that you are panting after exertion. You might feel short of breath lying in bed, especially when you are flat, and find that raising the head of your bed or using more pillows makes you comfortable. Sometimes you become breathless only in the middle of the night. Getting up and walking around sometimes helps. You may begin to notice that your legs are swelling, which is usually worse at the end of the day. This *edema* (swelling) can be so gradual that you may not be aware of it.

If you have not had a heart attack or rheumatic fever, you may not be aware that you have heart disease. Some people know only that they had high blood pressure for many years before the symptoms of chronic heart failure show up. If you begin to experience these symptoms, *heart failure* might be diagnosed. Your physician will usually do a number of tests, including a chest X-ray, an electrocardiogram, and certain blood tests. Treatment, often with a combination of medications, is usually successfull.

Like chronic heart failure, chronic *pulmonary breathlessness* progresses gradually, often occurring with a cough, excessive phlegm, or wheezing. Sometimes there are no symptoms other than the awareness that physical activity has become more difficult.

Shortness of breath from lung disease is more common if you were a smoker. This is by far the most common cause of chronic respiratory disease. Unfortunately, many people foolishly continue to smoke even though they know the connection between smoking and their symptoms. You may have had wheezing and coughing for many years, or other symptoms that signify the development of chronic bronchitis and emphysema.

As in heart failure, you may have some swelling in your legs, especially if the lung disease is severe. You may learn to partially close your lips as you walk which makes breathing seem easier, and notice your hands tend to be gray or blue. There is usually little tolerance for cold weather, which often aggravates breathlessness. Tests for these symptoms include a chest X-ray, an electrocardiogram, and pulmonary function tests, which allow the physician to determine the cause and extent of the lung damage and measure the response to treatment.

On rare occasions your physician may recommend a *lung biopsy*, in which a small piece of lung tissue is removed and examined under a microscope. This facilitates a diagnosis that may have been difficult to determine by other means.

Another condition that causes breathing difficulty is *pleural effusion* (an accumulation of fluid between the lung and chest wall). Often, the physician will remove this fluid to relieve symptoms and diagnose the reason for its accumulation. The causes include infections, inflammatory diseases, and tumors. *Thoracentesis* (removal of fluid) is usually painless and has very little risk.

Occasionally, a *pleural biopsy* may be necessary, in which a needle is inserted to remove a small piece of the *pleura* (lining of the chest wall). This is simpler than a lung biopsy, and it helps to clarify the cause of fluid accumulation.

Most people with chronic lung disease causing breathlessness can be helped if medical advice is followed. Stopping smoking is the single most important step you can take.

HEART PALPITATIONS

Heart palpitations are often the result of an excessively fast or irregular heart rhythm (cardiac arrhythmia). You will probably be aware of an irregular heartbeat, even if it lasts only a few seconds or minutes, and you may feel dizzy and fall. The palpitations may be infrequent or occur many times during the day. You might sense a "missed beat" or feel as though your heart has stopped. Some people experience a fluttering in the chest or "butterflies." In many older people the symptoms may be unclear, but they can be frightening. I have seen patients who have been found to have an irregular heart rhythm only after they have fallen and injured themselves.

It can be difficult at times to find the cause of palpitations. The usual electrocardiograms may not show the abnormal heart rhythm. A test using a Holter ambulatory monitor (ambulatory cardiograph) may be necessary to determine the exact cause of the palpitations. This is available in most medical centers. After diagnosis, the problem is usually treated successfully.

DIZZINESS AND FALLS

Many of us at some time have experienced dizziness. In the older person the symptoms may be a sense of spinning, unsteadiness, or falling. The causes of dizziness are many, but it results from a complicated upset of parts of the body that normally maintain your balance and steadiness.

One common cause of dizziness in older persons is disease affecting the balance mechanism of the inner ear. It may occur along with poor hearing or a ringing and buzzing in the head. Sometimes the blood supply to the balance mechanism is damaged. A commonly overlooked cause of dizziness is an irregular heartbeat (cardiac arrhythmia). This symptom may show itself as a feeling of lightheadedness or fainting, and it can result in repeated falls. You may not experience heart palpitations, which many physicians consider necessary in order to make this diagnosis. The same problems that lead to dizzy spells and palpitations may cause repeated falls. Your physician should carefully examine your heart rhythm to make sure that this is not the reason for your falls.

It is important to distinguish cardiac arrhythmias from other causes of dizziness. If your physician suspects an arrhythmia, he may have you carry a *Holter ambulatory monitor* (ambulatory cardiograph). During the period of the examination (usually twenty-four hours), you go about your normal activities and keep a diary of your symptoms.

One of the causes of dizziness is uneven control of blood pressure. Rising from a bed or chair may cause a large fall in your blood pressure and lead to a temporary decrease in the blood circulation to the brain. This can be aggravated by medications that you are taking for high blood pressure or for heart failure. Your blood pressure should be checked and measured while you are lying down and then once again when you are sitting and standing. You may find that your symptoms occur when you change your posture. It is very important to tell this to your doctor because this description may be the main clue to the correct diagnosis.

The causes of dizziness are often overlooked. Unfortunately, many physicians assume that when this symptom occurs in an older person it is always because of a poor blood supply to the balance mechanism. Since there is no effective treatment for this condition, patients may either not be treated at all or be put on medications such as aspirin or anticoagulants (blood thinners). Some physicians try antihistamines because some prevent the giddy sensation associated with motion sickness. They rarely give relief in the older person, however. Unless the cause for dizziness is found, your symptoms may go unrelieved.

Older people have a greater tendency to fall than younger people. But often it is assumed that they are more fragile and that falling is a natural consequence of aging. Although falls are common, the reasons are distinct from age alone. Obviously, a fall in an older person can be very dangerous. There is an increased tendency to break bones, and lacerations and head injuries are more common and more dangerous than in younger people.

The causes of repeated falls are often the result of an abnormality that usually can be treated. Your physician will have to examine you thoroughly in order to find out why you have fallen. All too frequently, only the injury caused by the fall is focused on. Among the reasons for falls are excessive changes in blood pressure, perhaps because of an underlying disease or because of medications that you are taking to treat heart failure or high blood pressure. Tranquilizers, sleeping pills, and antidepressants may also cause extreme lowering of the blood pressure.

Another common cause of falls is weakness of the legs. This sometimes follows brain damage that may have occurred as the result of a stroke that may not have been recognized. Your balance mechanism also can be impaired after a stroke or other disease affecting the brain.

Parkinson's disease, especially in its milder form, may not be recognized by your doctor or your family. You may have difficulty raising your legs properly and have a tendency to trip. A careful examination will usually reveal a degree of rigidity and stiffness of the muscles, which is characteristic of this disorder.

An elderly lady was sent to the hospital with a fractured hip. While she was being prepared for surgery, she told the orthopedic surgeon that she had fallen from a chair. When I spoke to her after the operation, she was not able to explain why she fell. She said, "I just found myself on the floor with a pain in my leg."

A few days later, a nurse found her collapsed in bed. By the time the doctor arrived, she had awakened. She eventually was found to suffer from episodes of an excessively slow heart rhythm *(bradyarrhythmia)*. A pacemaker was implanted to regulate her heart rhythm, and she experienced no further falls.

It is never enough to treat only the injury from a fall. Although you may describe your fall as "accidental," you should consult your physician so that he can determine the cause.

CHAPTER 8

Heart Disease

Older people frequently have specific symptoms and problems that are less vivid than in younger individuals with the same illness, and these can present a challenge to the physician. Also, drugs that are effective in younger people may be less well tolerated by an older person. A number of difficulties often affect the elderly at the same time, and each must be taken into consideration in order to receive proper treatment.

HOW THE HEART WORKS

The heart is a muscular pump that has a right side and a left side, each of which is divided into two chambers or compartments. The smaller compartment is called the *atrium* (or *auricle*) and the larger is called the *ventricle*. Blood flows through the *veins* and is channeled into the right atrium. From there it is pumped into the right ventricle.

The *lungs* receive the blood that is pumped *from* the right

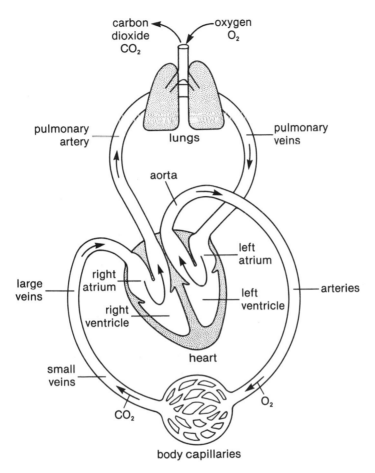

carbon dioxide CO₂

oxygen O₂

pulmonary artery

pulmonary veins

lungs

aorta

left atrium

right atrium

large veins

left ventricle

arteries

right ventricle

small veins

heart

CO₂

O₂

body capillaries

RELATIONSHIP OF HEART, LUNGS AND BODY.

ventricle. After passing through the lungs, the blood enters the left atrium and is then forced into the left ventricle. From here it is pumped into the *aorta*, the main artery from the heart, and then is directed through the smaller arteries to supply the needs of the whole body.

Each atrium is separated from the ventricles by one-way *valves* that prevent the blood from flowing backward from the atrium into the ventricle during contraction (pumping). Other valves prevent the blood from backing up from the lungs into the right ventricle and from the aorta into the left ventricle. These four valves, when healthy, assure that blood pumped by the heart always flows in a forward direction.

The blood that enters the right side of the heart through the right atrium is low in *oxygen* because it has passed through the body and transferred its oxygen supply to the tissues. In exchange for the oxygen, the muscles and organs produce *carbon dioxide*, a waste product that must be removed from the blood. The right ventricle therefore pumps blood that is low in oxygen and high in carbon dioxide to the lungs. Within the lungs the carbon dioxide is exhaled and oxygen-rich air inhaled and absorbed into the blood. From the lungs this oxygen-rich blood is delivered to the left atrium and passes into the left ventricle. The aorta receives the blood from the left ventricle, which works harder than the right ventricle and therefore has thicker muscular walls.

Your *heart muscle (myocardium)* requires its own nourishment and oxygen to work properly, and it has its own arteries that bring oxygen-rich blood to it from the aorta. These *coronary arteries* (blood vessels) bring blood to all the muscular compartments of the heart, thereby assuring their ability to keep pumping without interruption.

In addition to the muscle and valves, the heart has its own electrical system, which controls its function and assures that it pumps in a *regular rhythm.* It also assures that the atria and ventricles will pump in proper sequence. The heart also contains nerves, which can either speed up or slow down its rate. In a normal heart the rhythm is regular and the rate is appropriate for the demands made on it.

Both sides of the heart pump synchronously. Therefore, the same amount of blood that is pumped into the lungs during each heartbeat is also pumped into the aorta. If this balance is upset, blood can back up and collect in the lungs or in the body, thus upsetting the whole equilibrium. It is similar to an orchestra that would have the first and second violins playing at slightly different speeds. The sound would be awful, and one group would finish playing before the other.

Diseases of the heart can result from abnormalities of any of its parts. Quite often, the nourishment of the heart muscle is impaired because of disease affecting the coronary arteries that supply it. The heart's electrical system may become irregular, meaning the cardiac rhythm and speed will be abnormal. Also, the valves that separate the compartments may become damaged and either prevent blood from flowing smoothly and rapidly from one part of the heart to the other or cause it to backup. Veins and arteries going to and from the heart can also become diseased. Sometimes the heart muscle itself becomes abnormal and cannot pump effectively.

All of these disturbances can cause heart disease, and more than one problem may exist at the same time. In most instances a specific diagnosis can be made and effective treatment begun.

ANGINA PECTORIS

Angina pectoris is part of *ischemic heart disease*, which results from an impaired blood supply. At one end of the spectrum is angina pectoris; at the other end is *myocardial infarction*, also known as coronary thrombosis or "heart attack."

The blood supply to the heart can become impaired gradually, and this slow, progressive narrowing of coronary arteries by the buildup of fats in the blood vessel walls (*atherosclerosis*) usually leads to the symptoms of angina pectoris. The heart muscle receives less blood and is not able to work effectively. If the heart muscle is temporarily stressed beyond its ability to function properly because of the impaired blood supply, the pain of angina pectoris occurs.

In many ways an attack of angina pectoris is a warning that the heart is not getting enough blood. Some people think of it as a "cry for help" from a painful heart. Not everyone with angina pectoris develops a myocardial infarction, however. And not everyone who has a heart attack has had previous episodes of angina pectoris, which could have acted as a warning. An attack of angina pectoris is usually reversible if the demands of the heart are decreased by resting or taking medication. A myocardial infarction, on the other hand, means that part of the heart muscle has died because of lack of blood. In this situation other parts of the heart try to take on the work that the damaged heart muscle can no longer do.

Usually, the common symptoms of angina pectoris are a pressure, heaviness, ache, or pain behind the breastbone. The sensation often comes with exercise and is relieved by rest. You may feel the pain in places other than your chest: It can occur in one or both arms, especially the left arm, from the shoulder to the hand, or in the neck or jaw. Sometimes the pain goes through to the back, between the shoulder blades. Occasionally, the pain is felt so low in the chest that you may think it is indigestion.

You may notice the symptoms following a heavy meal or after eating something cold, such as ice cream. Some people are particularly aware of pain when they walk into a cold wind, and they often protect their face with a scarf to prevent an attack. Housework can cause attacks of angina pectoris that are not immediately recognized. There are many women who experience their first symptoms of angina pectoris while vac-uuming, a very stressful exercise, and do not complain to their physician because they think it is muscle strain from house-work.

Sexual activities may cause the symptoms of angina pectoris. Because of the circumstances, the discomfort may be confused with muscle tension and disregarded. Or because older people often have difficulty discussing their sexual activities with their physician, they may avoid disclosing the discomfort to him.

After a while the symptoms of angina usually fall into a

predictable pattern. The same type of activity or exercise brings on the distress. You may find that you can prevent the discomfort by avoiding those activities that usually cause the pain or rest as soon as it appears. Sometimes the symptoms are so mild that they are easily tolerated, and merely slowing down on physical exertion will relieve them.

How is the diagnosis of angina pectoris made?

To diagnose angina pectoris, your physician must carefully obtain your medical history. Sometimes the story is so unusual that the diagnosis may not be immediately evident. One elderly man complained of pain in his jaw, which occurred while eating, walking, and when he was sexually excited. He thought it was a toothache and visited a dentist, who refitted his dentures. However, this did not relieve his pain. On one occasion the "toothache" became so severe that he went to his doctor, who examined him and did an electrocardiogram. This revealed evidence of a prolonged angina attack. He was sent to the hospital, where treatment for angina thoroughly relieved his "toothache."

Some conditions can mimic angina, especially in the older person. These include diseases of the spine in the neck region. A *hiatus hernia*, with stomach acid regurgitating into the esophagus, also may be mistaken for angina.

Tests to diagnose angina include a physical examination with measurement of blood pressure, listening with the stethoscope to the chest and heart, examination of the pulse, and an *electrocardiogram*. Sometimes you may be given a *stress electrocardiogram*, where your heart is checked while doing increasing amounts of exercise. This shows electrocardiographic changes that suggest a decrease in your heart's blood supply, which may not be seen on the regular electrocardiogram. The test is not foolproof, but it can help confirm the diagnosis of angina pectoris in difficult cases.

How is angina pectoris treated?

After a diagnosis is made, your physician will prescribe medications. In addition, you can try to decrease the strain on your heart. If you are overweight, you should try to reduce. The less weight your heart has to carry, the less work it will have to do. If your blood pressure is elevated, your physician will probably recommend treatment. Lowering the blood pressure also decreases the amount of work the heart does. You must learn how to deal with emotional stress so that you do not get excited or upset easily. Some people benefit from an exercise program to improve the body's efficiency. This should be done only under careful supervision. It is usually necessary first to undertake other measures to improve your symptoms before starting on an exercise program.

The two main groups of medications used for the treatment of angina pectoris are *nitrates* and *beta-blockers*. The most commonly used nitrate is *nitroglycerin*, which has been available for many years. It should be taken whenever you experience an attack of pain or discomfort. In order to prevent attacks, you can take a tablet and allow it to dissolve under your tongue *before* you do something that you know always causes the pain of angina. This is often preferable to waiting for an attack to occur and then taking a nitroglycerin pill.

Nitroglycerin pills are effective *only* when they are allowed to dissolve under your tongue. They do not work when swallowed, and they deteriorate quickly if exposed to the air. You should store the tightly closed, unused bottle of pills in a dark, cool place, such as a refrigerator. If you have had nitroglycerin pills for more than a year, throw them away and get a new supply.

You will usually experience relief of discomfort from one or two pills within a few minutes. If you do not feel a tingling sensation under your tongue while the tablet is dissolving, it may mean that the pills are no longer active and you should get a new supply. If you do feel the tingling sensation and the pain is not relieved, it may mean that you are experiencing a more serious angina attack. In this situation go directly to a hospital emergency room.

Nitrates work in a number of ways. They cause the blood vessels in the body to dilate (expand), which decreases the work of your heart. They also allow some of the blood vessels in the heart to carry more blood, which improves the oxygen supply to the part of the heart that is affected. Because the blood vessels dilate, you may experience a headache or fullness in the head after you start taking nitrates. This can be very disturbing, especially if you have had problems with headaches before. Usually, if you decrease the amount of nitrate for a few days, the headaches will pass. You can then gradually increase the dose until you find relief of your anginal symptoms. Sometimes you may feel faint soon after you take the medication. To avoid this, take the first few doses while you are sitting or lying down.

The newer preparations of nitrates, called *long-acting* nitrates, include a very useful one known as *isosorbide dinitrate.* These medications can be swallowed, chewed, or allowed to dissolve under your tongue like nitroglycerin. Because their angina-relieving effect lasts for a few hours, they are usually prescribed to *prevent* attacks of angina, rather than after an episode has occurred. The medication should be taken every three or four hours, whether or not you are experiencing discomfort.

Nitroglycerin ointment is also prescribed for angina pain. A small amount applied to the skin is slowly absorbed over a few hours. It is especially useful before going to bed, if you are sometimes awakened with an attack.

The exact amount of nitrates and the combination of preparations required for each person is variable. Your physician will usually start with small doses and gradually increase them depending on the effect. Most people tolerate these medications well and get relief from their angina symptoms.

The second important group of drugs used to treat angina are *beta-blockers*, which act by blocking the effects of *adrenalin* on the heart. When you are under stress or have to undertake physical activity, your body produces adrenalin, which increases the heart's pumping speed and force. When the blood supply to the heart is impaired, the heart may not be able to respond to the effect of the adrenalin, and the symptoms of angina pectoris occur.

Many people produce excess adrenalin during periods of emotional stress or exercise, or when they are anxious. If this adrenalin is blocked from affecting the heart, attacks of angina pectoris that occur during these times can be prevented. However, for increased physical exertion, your heart has to augment its work. If this is completely prevented by the beta-blockers, you may find that you cannot do certain physical activities. Rather than experiencing an attack of angina pectoris, you may instead feel tired or even slightly faint. When this happens, you should slow down or stop what you are doing. You may notice that the medication slows your pulse, which indicates that it is working.

The beta-blockers are swallowed three or four times a day. Your physician will usually start with a small dose and gradually increase the amount depending on the degree of improvement. If you have a history of asthma or other lung disease, you may not be able to tolerate these durgs. The bronchi sometimes go into spasm and cause wheezing when these drugs are taken. Some of the new beta-blockers appear to be less likely to produce this side effect in the older person. The most common beta-blocker presently used is *propranolol* (Inderal®). Other, newer drugs are becoming available that may eventually replace propranolol; they have fewer side effects and can be taken less frequently. Your physician should examine the possible merits and dangers of the beta-blockers before beginning treatment. In general, if you tolerate them in small doses, you will not suffer from serious problems when the dose is increased.

With a combination of nitrates and beta-blockers, your anginal symptoms should be well controlled, and you can expect to experience little or no pain. You may find that, after starting treatment, you will be able to do more exercise than before. As symptoms improve, you may gradually increase your level of activity until you find the point at which symptoms return. You will then know your new limits of pain-free activity.

Heart surgery for the relief of anginal symptoms is less often considered in the older person than in the middle-age group in whom the illness occurs quite often and may threaten work and family life. However, as surgical techniques improve, the age limit will probably change. A number of medical centers already have effectively and successfully operated on older individuals who had not responded well to medical treatment. More results are necessary, however, before it is recommended that older people consider surgery.

HEART ATTACK
(MYOCARDIAL INFARCTION,
CORONARY THROMBOSIS)

Myocardial infarction is caused by a complete blockage of one of the coronary blood vessels that supplies blood to the heart muscle, resulting in a stoppage of the flow of oxygen-containing blood. A part of the heart muscle supplied by the blood vessel is irreversibly damaged because its oxygen and nutrient supply has been cut off. As a result, the heart's pumping action is disturbed. There are different degrees of heart attack, from mild to severe, depending on which coronary artery has been blocked and the amount of damage to the heart muscle. Most people who suffer from a heart attack survive it quite well. You can usually expect to return to a normal degree of activity after a period of convalescence.

What are the symptoms of a heart attack?

You may already know that you suffer from angina pectoris, and the pain experienced is similar. However, it is usually more severe and lasts longer, and it is *not relieved by rest or doses of nitroglycerin.* A heart attack can occur even if you have never experienced the pain of angina pectoris. You may suffer no pain at all and a routine electrocardiogram may show that you have had a so-called silent heart attack. This is more likely to happen if you suffer from diabetes mellitus.

Typically, the pain is felt behind the breastbone and is pressing or squeezing in nature. It often spreads to the neck and jaw and frequently down the arms or through to the back. You may have a feeling of fullness or heaviness in the lower part of the chest and upper abdomen, which is often mistakenly thought to be indigestion. It is not unusual to feel dizzy, vomit, and break out in a sweat. Shortness of breath often occurs, and some people feel as if they are choking.

What will happen in the hospital if a heart attack is suspected?

If you experience the symptoms of a heart attack, you should go directly to a hospital. Do not wait to speak to your doctor, and do not try to drive yourself to the hospital. Get there as soon as you can.

As soon as you arrive, you will probably be admitted to a special section of an emergency room and hooked up to a heart monitor that will show your heart's rate and rhythm. An electrocardiogram will be done to try to determine whether or not you have suffered from a heart attack. Blood tests and a chest X-ray will also be done to determine the extent of the heart damage and whether there are any complications.

You will be given medications such as *morphine*, which will relieve your pain. Most hospitals will then admit you to a special cardiac *intensive care unit.* You will again be hooked up to a monitor, which will continuously measure and record your heart rate and rhythm. You will also receive an intravenous infusion. This can be used to administer drugs to control abnormal heart rhythms or an excessively slow or fast heart rate, which can complicate a heart attack.

Other complications that can occur during the first few days after a heart attack include the accumulation of fluid in the lungs. This is called *heart failure* and may be a temporary consequence of a heart attack. If this occurs, you may receive *diuretics*, which will help remove the excess fluid from your lungs, improve your ability to breathe, and improve the pumping efficiency of your heart. *Digoxin*, used to improve the strength with which the heart works and to correct abnormal rhythms, may also be given.

During your time in the intensive care unit, you will have repeated electrocardiograms in order to measure the extent of heart damage. Blood tests that measure *cardiac enzymes* will also be done. These substances are normally found within healthy heart-muscle cells, but when the muscle is damaged, they leak into the blood. The quantity found determines the extent of the damage. As the attack finishes, the level of cardiac enzymes returns to normal.

Medications such as *nitrates* and *beta-blockers* may be given during the heart attack or through the recovery phase to try to decrease the extent of injury. Not everyone tolerates or benefits from these drugs at the time of a heart attack, however. These medications are often started after the attack, especially if there are symptoms of angina pectoris.

What can you expect after a heart attack?

If all goes well during the first few days, you will usually be allowed to get out of bed and sit in a chair. After five or six days you may be allowed to walk around your room. By this time you will probably have been transferred from the intensive care unit to a medical floor, where you will continue to recuperate. Most people require two to three weeks of total hospitalization if there were few complications. Some older people may require more time before they are strong enough to return home.

Following the hospital convalescence, you may return home if your environment is suitable. This depends on the number of stairs you have to climb or whether help is available. A convalescent home could be helpful if your progress has been slow. Over the next three or four weeks your activities can gradually be increased. Usually, you can return to your normal level of function in six to eight weeks. Most older people tolerate their first heart attack fairly well, and many have had more than one myocardial infarction without too much damage.

Following a heart attack, you may or may not suffer again from angina pectoris. This depends on the extent of heart damage. You may have no other symptoms or you may have so damaged your heart that you will require medications to support its ability to work properly. During the period of recuperation you should avoid putting excess strain on your heart. Walking should be done slowly initially and very gently and gradually increased.

After the attack you may require nitrates or beta-blockers. If you experienced heart failure during the attack, you may need digoxin and diuretics to keep the heart working at its best. If the heart rhythm becomes irregular during or after a heart attack, drugs may be necessary to correct the abnormality.

The fact that you can tolerate a heart attack extremely well is illustrated by an elderly man who told me that after his attack fifteen years before, a physician told him that he had only six months to live. That physician soon passed away and the patient found another doctor. About five years later the patient suffered a second heart attack. His second physician told him that he had anywhere from six months to a year to live. Later that year, the second doctor passed away and the patient continued with his activities without seeking a new physician.

At the time that I saw him he was in his late seventies and was feeling and functioning very well, although his electrocardiogram revealed evidence of his previous heart attacks. He asked me, "How long do I have to live?" I considered that the other two physicians died soon after they told him that he had from six months to a year, so I told him, "Anywhere from twenty to thirty years. I am not taking any chances!"

HEART FAILURE

Heart failure is a condition in which the ability of the heart to pump blood efficiently is impaired. Thus blood is not properly distributed throughout the body, and it backs up in the lungs. As the blood fills the lungs, the plasma (the fluid part of the blood) seeps into the air spaces and floods them. Oxygen cannot be taken into the congested lung and carbon dioxide cannot escape. This can cause shortness of breath and a choking sensation.

Heart failure can occur suddenly (acute heart failure) or gradually (chronic heart failure). Acute heart failure is the more frightening, whereas chronic heart failure may take a long time before you become aware of symptoms. Many people confuse heart failure with heart attacks. Although heart attacks can lead to heart failure, they are different illnesses.

What are the causes and symptoms of acute heart failure?

Acute heart failure is caused by a sudden impairment of the heart's pumping action. It most commonly affects the left side of the heart first although it can affect the right side or both sides simultaneously.

If the left ventricle suddenly fails to work effectively, the blood that it normally pumps to the body will back up into the lungs. This is called *pulmonary edema.* The most common causes of acute left-sided heart failure are heart attacks (myocardial infarction) and sudden abnormalities in heart rhythm.

During an episode of acute heart failure, you may suddenly feel very short of breath. If the heart failure is the result of a heart attack, you may first experience chest pain, although this does not always occur; if it is the result of an abnormality of your heart rhythm, you may first feel palpitations. Sometimes the attack occurs so quickly that the only symptom you feel is severe breathlessness. You may have difficulty lying down or finding a comfortable position sitting or standing. Sometimes you may have several attacks at night before you realize that something is seriously wrong.

What is the treatment for acute heart failure?

Acute heart failure is a medical emergency and treatment must be prompt. The medications include *diuretics*, which can be given intravenously (directly into the vein). The most common diuretic is *furosemide*. Many physicians carry this drug with them so that they can start emergency treatment even before you arrive at a hospital.

Digoxin, which increases the strength of the heart and also controls many types of irregular heart rhythms, is also often used intravenously. *Morphine* is given to decrease fear and anxiety, and it also helps to remove excess fluid from the lungs. Oxygen is usually given through a mask.

One of the older treatments for acute heart failure is *phlebotomy* (blood letting). During this procedure anywhere from 100 to 500 cc of blood may be removed from a vein through a needle. This procedure was used for many years after it was learned that removing blood improved the efficiency of the heart. As potent medications became available, the need for phlebotomy decreased. However, on occasion, acute heart failure that is difficult to treat medically might respond to phlebotomy. It is a painless procedure that can improve your condition dramatically, so there is no reason to fear it.

The treatment of acute heart failure, especially when there is pulmonary edema, is best carried out in hospital. X-rays, electrocardiograms, and blood tests are often needed to decide on the best therapy. If your physician sees you before going to the hospital, he may start treatment with furosemide and morphine to prevent the attack from getting worse before you arrive.

How dangerous is acute heart failure?

Depending on the underlying cause of the illness, the prognosis (the likely outcome) is usually good. Most individuals can be removed from immediate danger. If the cause of the heart failure is the result of severe, irreparable damage to the heart, such as in a massive heart attack, it may not respond to treatment and progress to *pump failure*. In this situation the pumping action of the heart is so impaired by heart muscle damage that therapy cannot improve its working action enough to fulfill the body's needs. This occurs rarely.

What causes chronic heart failure?

One of the common causes of chronic heart failure is *ischemic heart disease* (damage to the heart muscle caused by poor blood supply or previous heart attacks). Persistent high blood pressure or disease of the heart valves as occurs in rheumatic heart disease can also lead to chronic heart failure. Other diseases of the heart muscle, called *cardiomyopathies*, can also cause chronic heart failure and occur for many reasons, including alcoholism and inflammatory illnesses. On occasion, heart failure may be the result of an overactive or underactive thyroid gland (see page 358). Certain drugs can sometimes cause fluid to accumulate and aggravate heart failure.

What are the symptoms of chronic heart failure?

The usual symptoms of chronic heart failure are general tiredness and a decrease in the amount of activity that can be performed. Often sleeping becomes difficult, especially when you lie flat on your back. There may be some swelling of the legs and abdomen. If you gain weight that cannot be accounted for by increased food intake, it probably is the result of a gradual accumulation of fluid within your body. This also accounts for the swelling of the legs and abdomen.

How is the diagnosis made?

The diagnosis is made on the basis of your medical history and physical examination. The physician may find fluid accumulation in your body and evidence of decreased pumping action of your heart. Chest X-rays, electrocardiograms, blood tests, and other tests may be necessary to prove the diagnosis and explain the cause.

What is the treatment?

Although many drugs are effective, some general measures are useful in controlling chronic heart failure. A restriction of your salt intake may be very useful. Bed rest can help the heart do its work more efficiently and is helpful especially during the early stages of therapy.

Diuretics are often used to help the kidneys get rid of the extra fluid accumulation. By decreasing the amount of fluid in the body, your heart's pumping action becomes more efficient. *Digoxin* is also employed to improve the heart's pumping action and regulate some abnormal rhythms. You may benefit from a combination of a diuretic and digoxin. If hypertension (high blood pressure) plays a significant role in the cause of your heart failure, drugs, in addition to diuretics, can be used to lower the blood pressure. When the heart failure is the result of an abnormal heart rhythm, medications to control the rhythm may be effective.

When the heart suffers from a disease that decreases the speed of the heartbeat to a point where it can no longer efficiently pump blood, a pacemaker might be needed. This device ensures that the heart pumps fast enough to do its work.

An underactive or overactive thyroid gland can aggravate heart failure. Correction of the thyroid disorder makes the treatment of the heart failure easier. If you suffer from anemia, treatment may rectify the symptoms of heart failure.

Most older persons with chronic heart failure will improve with treatment. The long-term prognosis is generally good. The degree and duration of improvement depends on the underlying cause of the disease more than on the illness itself. If you are being treated for chronic heart failure, the single most effective way to determine whether the control is good is by weighing yourself regularly. Any significant weight gain is usually the result of fluid accumulation. This may occur long before the extra fluid becomes visible to you or your physician. If so, your physician will usually alter your drugs in order to improve the heart's function, and this should eliminate the extra fluid. Medication changes may be required every now and then to achieve smooth control.

CARDIAC ARRHYTHMIA (IRREGULAR HEARTBEAT)

The electrical conduction system of the heart normally assures that it beats in a regular rhythm, but a number of cardiac diseases disturb this process. Erratic heart rhythms are called *arrhythmias*. There are many types of heart arrhythmias, but they can be divided into *fast arrhythmias (tachyarrhythmia)* and *slow arrhythmias (bradyarrhythmia)*.

During an arrhythmia the amount of blood that the heart pumps to the body is decreased. Therefore, the brain gets less oxygen and nourishment than it needs. If the arrhythmia is serious or prolonged, you may become mentally confused or even lose consciousness. Usually, the symptoms are less severe and may be fleeting as the rhythm changes back to a normal, regular one.

What is a tachyarrhythmia (fast heartbeat)?

In this condition the heart begins to beat very quickly, either regularly or erratically. The speed may be so fast that its efficiency may be disturbed. You may feel a thumping or fluttering in your chest or symptoms such as dizziness, faintness, chest pain, or shortness of breath. The episode may be brief, occurring for only a few seconds or minutes, or it may last longer, until something is done to stop it. In many older people the attack occurs frequently, starting and stopping by itself. In others it may occur only once for an extended period and require medical attention to control it. You may have had an arrhythmia for many years and have become used to it, or the symptom may be new and therefore puzzling and frightening.

One elderly lady complained to me that she could feel her neck "jump" every few days. When she felt the jumping, she became short of breath and lacked energy. In her case the feeling in her neck was because one of the large arteries coming from the heart was beating at the very fast, irregular speed of her heart. She never felt palpitations. Treatment of her arrhythmia cured the sensation in her neck.

How is tachyarrhythmia diagnosed and treated?

One of the great difficulties in treating fast arrhythmias is that they may last momentarily, thereby making the diagnosis difficult to establish. In recent years the use of the Holter ambulatory monitor (twenty-four-hour electrocardiographic record) has helped physicians discover the various kinds of rhythms that may cause these symptoms. Sometimes the arrhythmia is more prolonged or constant and can be diagnosed by a physical examination and ordinary electrocardiogram.

In most cases the fast rhythm can be controlled with a single drug or a combination of drugs. One important drug is *digoxin*, which stabilizes the rhythm. Other *antiarrhythmics*, such as *quinidine* and the newer *beta-blockers*, may also be useful in some types of fast arrhythmias.

Usually, a physician will try one medication at a time to see if it is effective in controlling the rhythm. A second or third drug may be added until the correct combination is found. When

196

treatment is successful, symptoms will disappear or decrease. The physician can verify the success of therapy by repeating the electrocardiogram or the twenty-four-hour electrocardiographic tracing. These may show evidence of persistence of the arrhythmia, despite an abatement of symptoms, or they may confirm that the cause of the symptoms has been corrected.

Some fast rhythms are more dangerous than others. The physician will decide on the necessity of treatment by analyzing the underlying heart disease causing the abnormal rhythm and the likely result of therapy. In most cases an abnormal rhythm can be controlled and symptoms abolished.

What causes a bradyarrhythmia (slow heartbeat)?

Slow rhythms can occur during a heart attack, or spontaneously because of disease in the heart's electrical system. The symptoms are similar to the fast rhythm, although you will not feel palpitations or chest flutterings. However, you may experience dizziness, fainting, shortness of breath, and heart failure. An electrocardiogram or an ambulatory monitor may be needed to establish which type of slow rhythm is causing your symptoms. Like the fast rhythms, it may be permanent or transient.

Treatment might consist of changing medications or by installing a pacemaker. In most instances the slow rhythm can be effectively controlled and your symptoms will be relieved.

Do heart rhythms ever change from one to the other?

Your heartbeat may alternate between an excessively fast and a disturbingly slow rhythm. This condition is known as *tachy-brady syndrome*. The diagnosis is difficult to make and may require frequent examinations with an ordinary electrocardiogram or a twenty-four-hour electrocardiogram. Sometimes the disease may begin as a slow rhythm and progress to a fast rhythm and swing back and forth between.

Treatment may require a pacemaker to treat the slow rhythm and one or more antiarrhythmic drugs to control the fast rhythm.

PACEMAKERS

One of the newer technical marvels is the cardiac pacemaker, an electronic, battery-operated computer that can determine whether or not the heart is beating at a sufficiently fast speed. The computer is attached to a wire that is inserted through a vein to enter the heart. When the heart beats too slowly, the pacemaker electronically stimulates it to beat at the proper speed.

Pacemakers are inserted by heart surgeons. However, the decision to have one put in is usually made by a heart specialist (cardiologist). Usually, a number of electrocardiograms or ambulatory monitoring sessions are required before the decision is made to install one.

When is a pacemaker necessary?

One common disease affecting older individuals is *heart block.* The heart has its own electrical system to ensure that it pumps at a sufficient speed to meet the body's needs. Normally, the atrium beats first and helps the blood enter the ventricle, which then pumps it to the body. Electrical impulses tell the atrium and ventricle when to beat.

A number of illnesses affect the heart and interfere with this electrical system. The stimulating impulses that would normally cause the heart to increase its speed according to the body's demands may not reach the heart muscle. The message to pump faster is therefore blocked. Under these circumstances you may suffer from attacks of fainting or dizziness. You may develop heart failure, which cannot be treated adequately because the drugs required may slow the heart rate excessively. The pacemaker overcomes the block, speeds up the heart, and allows it to function effectively.

Is it difficult to install and maintain a pacemaker?

Pacemakers are no more than two-and-a-half inches round and half an inch thick. Smaller, lighter models are becoming available. A pacemaker is implanted under the skin in the region of the upper front part of the chest. The operation takes from thirty to sixty minutes. The wire is threaded through a vein into the right ventricle.

There is virtually no danger in having a pacemaker implanted, and rarely do complications arise. Sometimes infections occur that require its removal, or defects in some models are discovered. When this occurs, the device is changed.

If you have a pacemaker, you will require follow-up examinations to make sure that it is working properly. This is usually arranged through a pacemaker clinic at the hospital where the pacemaker was implanted. Many clinics have an arrangement whereby you can use your telephone to test the pacemaker. A small attachment is put over the pacemaker, and the electrical messages are sent by telephone to the clinic. About five to six years after insertion, most of the newer pacemakers need a battery change. The clinic will usually notify you of this after checking the effectiveness of the pacemaker.

You may have difficulty accepting the need for a pacemaker, especially if you have been relatively well and have never had surgery. You may be reluctant to have heart surgery and may not understand that your symptoms of fainting, dizziness, or heart failure may be because of a condition that can be easily treated. I have had difficulty at times trying to convince an older patient that a pacemaker would be of value. I recall one man who, despite frequent fainting spells, refused the device. I asked him if he had ever owned a car. He answered, "Of course, a

Buick." I remarked that that was a very good car, and he agreed. I asked him if the battery ever went dead. He looked at me quizzically and said, "Sure, you always have to change a battery sometime." I asked him if, instead of changing the battery, he had ever thought of throwing the car away. He responded, "That would be stupid to throw a good car away because it needs a battery." I answered, "Exactly." He agreed to have the pacemaker inserted, and he was still well three and a half years after this conversation—and had had no more fainting spells.

Another man in his late eighties came from England to Canada to see his relatives. During a family dinner he fainted and was brought to the emergency room, where he was found to have a very slow pulse. A pacemaker was inserted and he was able to continue his visit and then return to England. For the next two years he returned to Canada for family visits, and on each occasion he came to my office for an examination, where I found him to be extremely well. Recently, after four years, he required the battery to be changed. His physician in England informed me that now at the age of 90 the man had just returned from the Middle East, where he went to visit other members of his family. He is vigorous and active, thanks to his pacemaker.

VALVULAR HEART DISEASE

There are four valves in the heart, two of which separate the atria from the ventricles on both sides of the heart. The other two separate the large blood vessels that receive blood from the right and left ventricles. Proper heart function requires the smooth, coordinated working of these valves. They prevent the blood from traveling backward from the ventricle to the atrium or from the aorta and pulmonary artery to the ventricle. In other words, they assure the proper direction and flow of blood to the lungs and body.

Do older people suffer from valvular heart disease?

Valvular heart disease is most common in young people, either because of *congenital* (existing from the time of birth) problems or following illnesses such as rheumatic fever. Acute rheumatic fever usually occurs in children and young adults. It rarely occurs for the first time in an older person. However, the long-term effects of childhood rheumatic fever may have damaged your heart valves and impaired their function without you being aware of it. You may not recall that you ever had rheumatic fever and be surprised when you are told that you have rheumatic heart disease. At the time you may have had this illness, the basis for diagnosis was much less exact than now and often it was overlooked. Therefore, you can show evidence of a previously damaged heart valve for the first time in your later years.

In older people the most common cause of an abnormal valve is improper function of the muscles that control it or degenerative valve changes that can occur with age. If you have suffered a heart attack, you may have damaged the muscles that control the closure of the *mitral valve*, which separates the left atrium from its ventricle. In this instance your physician may hear a *heart murmur*, which means the valve is leaking. The amount of leakage is variable and depends on the extent of damage to the valve's supporting muscles.

In many elderly people heart murmurs can be heard even when there is no evidence of heart disease. These murmurs are often the result of the degeneration of a valve that does not necessarily affect its proper operation. You should not become upset if your physician hears a murmur, especially if he has not examined you previously. Unless there are new symptoms that suggest a change in heart function, these murmurs do not necessarily mean heart damage.

Your physician should record the type of murmur so that on further examinations he can see if it has changed. If he feels that your murmur is the result of rheumatic heart disease or that the murmur means poor function of the valve, he may make some recommendations about the possibility of surgery or the use of antibiotics to prevent bacterial endocarditis.

When is heart-valve surgery necessary?

In younger people some types of valvular problems are treated with open-heart surgery to replace the diseased valves. This is less often done in the older person because usually the risk of surgery far outweighs the potential benefit in terms of life expectancy. As surgical techniques improve and as life expectancy increases, many surgeons will probably become less reluctant to replace heart valves in older people. This has already occurred in some medical centers, and the results have been gratifying. In some older people heart surgery for valve replacement can be beneficial, so it should not be discounted without a thorough discussion with a cardiologist.

What are the dangers from a leaking heart valve?

More pertinent to you than heart surgery is the danger that your leaking heart valve might become infected and result in *bacterial endocarditis.* This happens if bacteria enter the bloodstream, adhere to a deformed valve and begin to multiply and spread to other parts of the body. If you have a defective heart valve, remind your physician and dentist so that you receive antibiotics before any surgery or dental treatment.

What types of heart surgery
are done on older people?

In general, heart surgeons are somewhat reluctant to do open-heart surgery for valvular or coronary artery disease on older people.

But great strides have been made in cardiac surgery. The *coronary bypass* procedure for angina pectoris and other forms of *ischemic heart disease* has become well developed. Most medical centers now perform this surgery, and thousands of patients have benefited from it. Newer surgical measures that are safer for the elderly are being developed.

The degree of success of coronary artery surgery is still not completely determined for all age groups. In the older patient the relative risks of surgery compared to medical treatment (using medications alone) have not yet been completely settled. It is known that you might get along for many years with angina pectoris in a state of relative comfort and carry out your normal activities without coronary bypass surgery. Some older people, of course, have died from coronary heart disease, and the question is often asked, "Would surgery have helped?"

As surgical techniques improve and as the advantages of surgical therapy become better defined, we may see more older people accepted for this kind of surgery. At present it is a controversial matter. Some surgical centers will consider you for coronary bypass surgery if your general health is good and if the tests, including a coronary *angiogram* (X-ray of the blood vessels to the heart), show that surgery is likely to be beneficial.

The decision must be made by you, using the advice of a cardiologist, who is well versed in the risk factors of such surgery. It should be done only in medical centers that have wide experience with older patients.

CHAPTER 9

Vascular (Blood Vessel) Disease

The vascular system, meaning the blood vessels, includes *arteries*, which bring blood from the heart *to* the various parts of the body, and *veins*, which return this blood to the heart after the nutrients and oxygen have been removed. Some diseases disturb the blood vessels alone, and others interact to affect both the blood vessels and the heart. Some illnesses affect the large vessels, whereas others affect the small ones. Some blood vessel diseases are generalized: Every organ and tissue of the body may be affected at the same time. One important condition that leads to widespread damage from diseased arteries is *atherosclerosis*.

ATHEROSCLEROSIS

Atherosclerosis is often loosely called *hardening of the arteries.* It is assumed by most people, including some physicians, that it is a natural consequence of aging. However, this disease is common in all age groups. During the Korean War it was found that many young American soldiers killed in battle had early signs of atherosclerosis. In contrast, older people from less advanced countries may reach their mature years with little evidence of this disorder.

The arteries normally have a very smooth lining, which allows blood to flow quickly and easily. In atherosclerosis the smooth lining becomes roughened and fatty material collects. As these deposits accumulate, calcium may also collect. Sometimes the deposits of fat and calcium become dislodged, leaving an uneven surface on the lining of the arteries. They gradually narrow the arteries, thereby interfering with the flow of blood. If the deposits become large enough, they may completely block the arteries and cut off the supply of oxygen- and nutrient-rich blood. This can cause severe damage or death to the tissues or organ supplied by that artery. If the atherosclerotic aggregate develops an irregular surface, the blood may clot within the arteries. This is called *thrombosis*, and it can cause a serious or fatal illness.

Another condition, called *arteriosclerosis*, is similar to athero sclerosis. However, the lining of the artery is not damaged in the same way as in atherosclerosis. Arteriosclerosis is the result of persistently high blood pressure. In many cases, however, prolonged high blood pressure causes further damage, and the artery eventually develops atherosclerosis.

Any artery in the body can be affected by atherosclerosis, but it most frequently affects larger blood vessels, such as those going to the heart, brain, and kidneys. The main artery, the *aorta*, often becomes diseased with atherosclerosis. Depending upon the vessel involved, the results may include heart attacks, strokes, kidney damage and aneurysms. The exact cause of atherosclerosis is not clear, but it is more common in Western society and less so in primitive cultures. Immigrants coming to the West from less developed countries often develop athero-sclerosis within a short period, just like the native inhabitants.

Among the influences that seem to increase the incidence of

atherosclerosis are diet, smoking, high blood pressure, diabetes mellitus, stress, and a lack of exercise. Probably a combination of many influences puts people in Western countries at special risk.

Measures to try and decrease the likelihood of atherosclerosis include alterations in diet. It seems that large amounts of animal fats have a deleterious effect on its development. Therefore, by increasing nonsaturated vegetable fats and oils and decreasing the intake of animal fat, you may be able to reduce the progression of this disease. The exact place of cholesterol, an animal fat, is still not completely clear. In general, however, you should limit the amounts of animal fat in your diet.

Other dietary influences include the amounts of refined sugar in your diet. Some authorities suggest that this excess carbohydrate increases the risk of atherosclerosis. Some physicians maintain that increasing the amounts of fiber in your diet can retard the development of atherosclerosis. Proof is difficult, however, because so many other factors seem to play a role.

There is no question that cigarette smoking has a major aggravating effect on the development of atherosclerosis. If you smoke, you have a greater risk of developing this disease at a younger age. If you suffer from diabetes mellitus, atherosclerosis may progress more quickly than if you were free from this disease. There seems to be a relationship between the degree of care with which the diabetes is controlled with diet and medications and the speed with which atherosclerosis develops. Therefore, if you have diabetes mellitus and are careless with your diet and also smoke, you are tempting fate.

It appears that people who become easily stressed develop atherosclerosis more quickly than those who are more relaxed. This is difficult to prove because people express their stress and emotions in different ways. However, it appears that tense, hard-driving individuals are more likely to develop atherosclerosis.

Women who are still menstruating are less likely to develop

atherosclerosis than those who have already gone through menopause. However, as more and more women smoke, this advantage appears to be lost. The later your menopause, the greater the lag in your development of atherosclerosis.

If you have *high blood pressure (hypertension)*, you are at greater risk. The less well this is controlled, the more rapidly the disease develops. It is essential, therefore, to follow your physician's advice and carefully maintain your medication therapy and limit your salt intake.

The many factors known to aggravate the development of atherosclerosis interact with your hereditary makeup. If you are lucky enough to have a family in which this disease is not common or develops late, you should use this good fortune to its best advantage. Avoid the risk factors that enhance the production of the atherosclerotic process. Do not smoke, follow a sensible diet, and exercise regularly. If you suffer from diabetes mellitus or hypertension, make sure that you treat them carefully.

HYPERTENSION (HIGH BLOOD PRESSURE)

Blood pressure is the force inside the blood vessels with which the blood is pumped. Each time the heart beats, it propels blood into the main artery (aorta) and from there through all the arteries of the body. The amount of pressure in the blood vessels determines whether the blood will reach all the organs efficiently. If the pressure is too low, the tissues of the body may suffer from lack of oxygen and nutrients. If the pressure is too high, the blood vessels and heart become damaged.

High blood pressure has been recognized for many years as being dangerous, although the cause is still not completely clear. Many factors contribute to it, including heredity, certain diseases, and diet. The large amounts of *salt* in Western diets is probably one factor in its increased frequency.

Uncontrolled high blood pressure takes its toll by causing

damage to your heart and blood vessels. Normally, blood vessels are flexible and can react to the increased pressure. As hypertension persists, they may become less resilient and eventually develop the fatty deposits of atherosclerosis. The vessel walls may become weakened and rupture or become blocked by fatty deposits and blood clots. When either hemorrhage into an organ or blockage of a blood vessel occurs, vital oxygen and nutrients cannot reach the tissues supplied by the blood vessels. The heart is also affected by high blood pressure. It must work harder to drive the blood through the body. If the pressure remains elevated for many years, your heart may weaken, and eventually you may develop heart failure.

Blood pressure is measured with a *sphygmomanometer*, a device that consists of an inflatable cuff that is wrapped around the arm. As the cuff expands, the arteries within the arm are compressed and the blood flow through them is blocked. The physician then listens with his stethoscope over an artery and gradually decreases the cuff pressure. The blood pressure is read on a scale. He first notes the pressure when he initially hears the blood trickling through the artery. This is the upper reading. As the cuff further deflates, the noises change and he determines the lower reading of the blood pressure. The *systolic* pressure (the upper number) is the highest level and the *diastolic* pressure (the lower number) is the lowest.

What does it mean if your blood pressure is high?

There is no longer any question that in younger people the diagnosis and proper treatment of hypertension can decrease the severe complications that may occur with advancing age. The danger of strokes and heart disease is greatly reduced when a younger person's high blood pressure is reduced to normal limits. For this reason, large screening programs have been instituted in the community, in hospital clinics, and by physicians to alert people who may have high blood pressure.

In the elderly blood pressure tends to become elevated

gradually. It has not yet been completely determined what levels may be normal for older individuals. We do not know exactly at what stage the risk of strokes and heart disease increases. Some studies suggest that blood pressure levels of greater than 160–180 systolic and 90–100 diastolic place older individuals at a greater risk of hypertensive complications.

Many physicians were taught that you may need the excessive blood pressure to pump blood through arteries that have become narrowed as part of the aging process. This now appears to be erroneous and has resulted in little effort being put into finding older people with hypertension and less effort being expended in their treatment. The picture is somewhat confusing for both the physician and you. Neither he nor you may be certain what should be done about a level of blood pressure that, if found in a younger person, would merit drug therapy. It also used to be taught that only a raised diastolic (lower) blood pressure was significant in causing the complications of hypertension. It has now been shown that in younger people a raised systolic (upper) pressure is also important. It is not certain whether this effect can be completely translated to the older individual, however.

Older people often have raised *systolic* blood pressures because of the loss of elasticity of their large blood vessels. This does not necessarily mean that the smaller blood vessels going to the brain, heart, and kidneys are abnormal. Your physician may find himself in a difficult situation if your systolic blood pressure is high, but your diastolic pressure is normal. He may judiciously try to lower your systolic blood pressure without excessively decreasing your diastolic level.

We do not yet know whether trying to reduce this elevated systolic blood pressure is worthwhile. Whether an 80 year old with a blood pressure of 220/90 will benefit from medications to lower the systolic level is difficult to establish. Most of the studies of the younger population to prove the benefits of treatment have taken ten to twenty years to accomplish. Some researchers, however, have shown that those older people who have already suffered from strokes and heart disease have higher levels of systolic and diastolic blood pressure. This information suggests that carefully lowering the blood pressure at *any* age is beneficial.

How is high blood pressure treated?

In general, I recommend that attempts be made to lower your blood pressure if it is consistently elevated above 170–180/ 95–100. You should try to reduce your weight and salt intake before taking drugs. In some people this, combined with a regular exercise program, is successful in lowering high blood pressure. If these measures are not enough, medications are necessary.

Your physician should check the effect of the antihypertensive (blood-pressure-lowering) treatment every few weeks in the early stages of therapy. Blood pressures should be measured with you sitting and standing. An excessive drop in blood pressure when you change position is usually a sign that the amount of medication should be decreased until your pressure returns to a safer level.

What medications are used to treat high blood pressure?

One type of medication often prescribed first to control high blood pressure is a *diuretic*. This allows excess salt and water to be passed by your kidneys. Diuretics alone may sufficiently lower your blood pressure to acceptable levels without additional medications. There are many types of diuretics, including a group known as *thiazides*, which induce your kidneys to pass excess potassium. Other diuretics, such as *spironolactone* and *triamterene*, often combined with thiazides, are also effective and tend to retain potassium.

A second group of drugs are the *beta-blockers*, which are also used to treat heart disease. They lower the blood pressure by affecting its control at various points, including the brain, heart, and kidneys. An older person may not always be able to tolerate these medications, but many varieties are suitable, and more are being developed.

Other medications affect the blood vessels themselves, and some also affect the brain's control of blood pressure. Drugs such as *alphamethyldopa* (Aldomet®) and *hydralazine* (Apresoline®) fall into this category.

Are there any side effects in the treatment of high blood pressure?

Although the drugs used to treat high blood pressure can be very effective, numerous side effects may be encountered. If you become dizzy or faint while taking these medications, it may mean that your blood pressure is dropping too low. And they may have an ill effect on your kidneys. This can be checked by measuring the levels of *urea* and *creatinine*, the body's normal waste products, in your blood. If the *uric acid* concentration becomes elevated, you may experience an attack of gout. Your blood sugar may rise and, if you have diabetes mellitus, this becomes more difficult to control.

Some older people become sleepy or mentally confused when they take medications to control high blood pressure. One of the important side effects of certain medications is impotence. This should not be attributed to your age, especially if it occurs after you start taking antihypertensive drugs. The loss of potassium from diuretics may make you feel weak, but this can be treated by increasing the citrus fruits and bananas in your diet or taking a potassium supplement.

These problems should be kept in mind when elevated blood pressure is being treated. If you feel ill, report the symptoms to your physician.

Is high blood pressure curable?

Even though antihypertensive (blood-pressure-lowering) treatment controls your blood pressure, it will never cure it. High blood pressure is curable only in some rare instances, such as when a tumor which produces excess amounts of adrenaline is surgically removed.

You may misunderstand your physician's delight that your blood pressure has returned to normal and stop your medications because you think you have been cured. But the next time you see your physician, your blood pressure may once again be elevated and you will not understand why. Neither will your physician unless you tell him that you have stopped taking or have adjusted your medication. In most cases high blood pressure can be controlled with drug therapy and general dietary measures. Discontinuance of the drugs will cause it to return to the elevated level, with all the dangers that accompany untreated high blood pressure. *Never stop your pills or modify the quantities you take until your physician tells you to.*

PERIPHERAL VASCULAR DISEASE

The blood vessels are lined with a smooth layer of cells that allows the blood to flow evenly and without interference. Atherosclerosis roughens this lining with collections of fatty material and calcium. If a blood vessel is affected by atherosclerosis, it can become partially or completely blocked. This can lead to problems in the tissues it supplies. When the lower aorta or the blood vessels going to the legs become diseased with atherosclerosis, the illness is called peripheral vascular disease.

What are the symptoms of peripheral vascular disease?

A common symptom is *intermittent claudication* (recurrent pain in lower limbs after exercise). This causes pain in your legs while walking or running, which is relieved when you rest. The blood supply to the legs is insufficient because the arteries are partially blocked. You may find that while walking you suffer discomfort in your buttocks or calves, and you might have to stop until the pain goes away. Thus you might alter your activities to avoid pain. In general, a certain amount of effort will always result in pain. In many ways the condition is similar to angina pectoris. Instead of a coronary artery being partially blocked in the heart causing the pain, an artery to your leg is blocked and the limb suffers the discomfort.

In some instances an artery becomes suddenly blocked completely as the result of a blood clot (thrombus), and the limb receiving blood through that artery becomes endangered. In such cases emergency surgery is required in order to remove the blockage and reestablish a sufficient blood supply to keep the limb alive. The surgery is often successful. However, when it is not, it may mean the loss of a limb.

Are medications helpful in the treatment of peripheral vascular disease?

The most important treatment is to prevent atherosclerosis. The measures that you take before the disease has advanced are more effective than treatment introduced after the damage has been done. However, a number of drugs are used to treat peripheral vascular disease. Some, known as *vasodilators*, can improve the blood supply to the skin of the affected limb, but they may inadvertently decrease the blood supply to the muscles. Although you may feel less pain when you take these medications, their effect is temporary. They do not reverse the underlying problem. Some physicians recommend anticoagulants (blood thinners) to decrease the likelihood of blood clots forming. This treatment may prevent further deterioration of the limb's poor blood supply. Aspirin and similar drugs that decrease the stickiness of blood are also used for this purpose. Their use is controversial and should be supervised by a physician.

In recent years there has been a great deal of discussion

about the effect of vitamin E on peripheral vascular disease. However, although some people report such an improvement in their symptoms that surgery can be avoided or postponed, it has not been proven that vitamin E actually works. Nevertheless, some physicians do recommend its use, especially in the older person for whom surgery appears to be excessively dangerous.

Is there any surgical treatment for peripheral vascular disease?

If you suffer from severe intermittent claudication, an attempt is usually made to show the extent of artery blockage. It is important to determine whether the blockage is *local* (at one spot in the blood vessel) or *diffuse* (affecting many areas simultaneously). If the blockage is limited to one area, and if the remainder of the blood vessel going to the limb is patent (not obstructed), a *bypass* operation may be done. The blocked area of the blood vessel is bypassed by the insertion of either a vein (taken from another part of the body) or an artificial graft (using synthetic material). This can be done quite successfully, and it is being performed more and more in older people as techniques improve and as beneficial results become clear. The relative risk of surgery must be weighed against the potential benefits. This often depends on your general health. If you have severe heart disease as well as peripheral vascular disease, the risk could be too great. You must also consider the amount of activity that you would like to do and how greatly the blockage limits your ability to do it. If, for instance, you rarely walk enough to experience pain, surgery may not be so important.

Sometimes small pieces of the atherosclerotic blood vessel become dislodged and cause a blockage of arteries in the feet or toes. This can lead to a total loss of blood supply and probable gangrene. This situation might also benefit from a bypass operation, which will improve the blood supply and allow sufficient nutrients to reach the affected area. In some cases, when correction is impossible, amputation of the affected limb may be necessary to prevent the progress of gangrene.

Are other treatments available?

A physician may recommend a *sympathectomy* for intermittent claudication due to peripheral vascular disease. In this minor operation, a surgeon cuts small nerves that regulate the carrying capacity of the blood vessels going to the limb. When the nerves are cut, the artery dilates (enlarges) and more blood reaches the leg. In some cases the improvement in blood supply relieves the painful symptoms enough to avoid bypass surgery. Sometimes a combination of a sympathectomy and bypass surgery is necessary to improve the blood supply to the limbs and ensure their function.

ANEURYSMS

An aneurysm is a swelling in one part of a large blood vessel that is caused by a weakening of its wall. As the pressure within the blood vessel pushes against the weakened area, the wall bulges out more and more, until it begins to look like a balloon. This causes the artery's wall to become even thinner and weaker. The most common blood vessel affected by an aneurysm is the aorta, the main blood vessel from the heart. It can occur anywhere along the aorta's passage through the chest and abdomen. Aneurysms can also occur less often in other arteries, such as those supplying the brain and kidneys.

Is an aneurysm dangerous?

In many cases there may be no symptoms of an aortic aneurysm until it begins to leak or burst. You may have no reason to seek medical advice until you notice a pulsating feeling within the abdomen. In most instances a physician discovers the aneurysm during a routine physical examination or during X-rays that are done for other reasons.

Aneurysms gradually become larger over a period of years. The leaking or bursting of an aneurysm, which causes sudden and rapid hemorrhage within the chest or abdomen, can be fatal.

Should surgery be performed on aortic aneurysms?

It may be difficult to decide whether you should have an aortic aneurysm removed and replaced with a synthetic graft to prevent it from leaking or rupturing. If you are in good health and the aneurysm is of sufficient size, it is better to have it removed before it leads to problems. With modern techniques, the benefits of elective surgery outweigh the risks in most healthy older people. However, if you have other medical problems and if your general health is poor, the risks may be too great. If the aneurysm is leaking or expanding quickly, emergency surgery is necessary. (The size of an aneurysm is measured with an *echogram*.) It is less likely for the older person to survive a ruptured aneurysm.

The symptoms of leakage may be vague but are usually those of pain. Depending on the location of the aortic aneurysm, the pain may be in the chest or abdomen and can be confused with a myocardial infarction (heart attack) or an abdominal illness. Frequently, there is back discomfort, which might be confused with other causes of back pain. If you have an aortic aneurysm without symptoms and surgery has not been recommended, you should go directly to a hospital in the event of a sudden onset of unexplained pain. Frequent follow-up examinations are mandatory if surgery for an aneurysm has not been done.

VARICOSE VEINS

Varicose veins occur when the valves which control the direction of flow in the veins of the legs leak and allow blood to collect. This results in the stretching and ballooning of the vein, which is often seen or felt as small bumps on the legs.

Many people who have had varicose veins for many years have received treatment with injections or surgery. Others have never received treatment, either because they were afraid or because the varicose veins were not a problem.

What problems are caused by varicose veins?

The most common consequences of varicose veins in the older person is an uncomfortable swelling of the legs and feet. In some instances blood clots (thrombosis) form within varicose veins, which can lead to severe pain and infection. Occasionally, a blood clot becomes dislodged and passes to the lungs, resulting in an embolism.

What treatment is available?

For the most part, treatment does not require surgery. One important measure, however, is to lose weight, which usually makes varicose veins more manageable.

You may benefit from small doses of *diuretics* to decrease the swelling. In general, these drugs should be avoided or used sparingly because, although the swelling may improve, dizziness and an excessive lowering of blood pressure can result.

The main purpose of therapy is to increase the outside pressure on the veins, thereby improving their ability to empty the pooled blood in the legs back to your circulation. In most cases elastic support stockings are sufficient. The stockings should go above the knees and should not have a tight band on the top, which could block the blood flow through the veins. In difficult cases some commercial companies will custom-make a stocking that will distribute the pressure evenly. For most people a standard elastic stocking from a surgical supply store is sufficient. Your doctor should check it to ensure that it fits well. It is best to put it on in the morning before you get out of bed, when your legs are not swollen.

Avoid standing in one position for a long time, and raise your legs whenever you are seated. If you must make a long trip, wear support stockings and exercise your leg muscles frequently. In a train or plane, get up and walk around. If you must sit for a long time in a car or bus, move your feet up and down in a rocking motion.

What complications can occur with varicose veins?

Sometimes, following an injury, you may develop a *varicose ulcer* as a result of a back-up of blood and fluid. In such a case, the tissues surrounding the vein become damaged and fail to heal adequately. In addition to an ulcer there may be severe external bleeding from the injured vein. This can be very frightening because the bleeding does not stop easily. If this occurs, raise your leg and apply firm pressure to the area until the bleeding stops. See a doctor as soon as possible. Because varicose ulcers take a long time to heal, prolonged bed rest or even hospitalization may be required. Occasionally, a skin graft to the ulcer might be necessary to speed healing.

PHLEBITIS

Phlebitis, another complication of varicose veins, occurs when the stagnant blood within a ballooned vein clots and causes a blockage. In many cases it is accompanied by inflammation or infection, which is often painful. Depending on the severity, hospitalization and treatment with anticoagulants, antibiotics, and antiinflammatory drugs is necessary. In mild cases treatment can be successfully carried out at home.

How can phlebitis cause lung damage?

If one of the blood clots breaks off from the vein, it will travel to the heart and lungs and cause a *pulmonary (lung) embolism.* The symptoms include chest pain, severe shortness of breath, heart palpitations, the coughing up of blood, and fluid in the lungs. Treatment with anticoagulants can prevent further clots from forming.

This condition is extremely dangerous. It occurs most often after long periods of bed rest, such as after surgery or during a prolonged illness. The best way to prevent it is to exercise your feet and legs frequently. The sooner you start walking after surgery or an illness, the less likely you are to develop a thrombosis or embolism.

CHAPTER 10

Respiratory Disease

Air enters the respiratory system through the nose and mouth. In the nose it is warmed and filtered by a lining of many small hairs. Large particles are kept out of the lungs by a *cough reflex*, which prevents them from entering the upper part of the *larynx* (voice box) or *trachea*. From the trachea, air passes through the large *bronchi* to the smaller bronchi, or *bronchioles*, which are covered with thousands of small hairs, or *cilia*. These constantly brush back any particles or bacteria that have passed through the throat and trachea. The cells also normally produce small amounts of *mucus*, a sticky substance that traps small particles and facilitates their easy removal from the bronchi. The bronchi become smaller and smaller and eventually lead into *alveoli* (air sacks of the lungs), where oxygen and carbon dioxide are exchanged in the blood.

The lining of the chest wall and lungs, called the *pleura*, is separated by the *pleural space*. During certain illnesses fluid collects in this space and separates the two sides of the pleura, causing the lung to become compressed. The chest wall contains bones (ribs and spine) and muscles, including the dia-

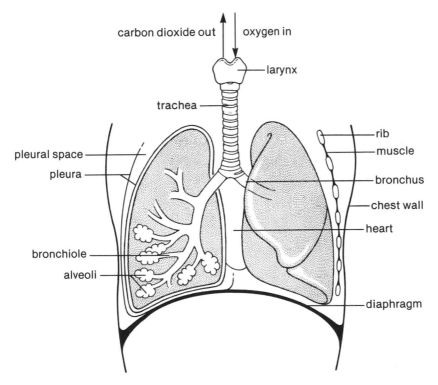

RESPIRATORY SYSTEM.

phragm (muscle separating the chest and abdomen). When air is inhaled, the chest expands; when it is exhaled, the chest contracts. Normally, the cycle of breathing occurs approximately twelve times a minute. Some diseases make breathing difficult or painful and result in shortness of breath.

UPPER RESPIRATORY INFECTIONS AND ALLERGIES

As air enters the upper respiratory tract—the nose, mouth, and sinuses—it is warmed and filtered before entering the lower respiratory system through the larynx and trachea. The lining of the upper part of the system protects the respiratory tract from infection and damage, although it can itself become infected by bacteria or viruses or occasionally develop an irritation, or *allergy*, to certain substances.

Are colds more dangerous in the elderly?

There is an old saying that a cold will improve in seven days with a doctor and in a week without. Usually colds are no more dangerous in older people than in younger ones. In people with heart or lung diseases, a cold may reduce the body's resistance and result in bacterial infections that can lead to bronchitis or pneumonia. This happens infrequently in a healthy elderly person.

Other than a mild analgesic, such as aspirin or acetaminophen, and plenty of hot fluids, there is little need to take medication for a cold. In fact, some over-the-counter medications taken to treat a cold may be more risky than the cold itself. Some people believe that large doses of vitamin C taken at the onset of a cold reduce its severity and duration. Whether or not this is true is unclear, but little harm will come from taking it.

Viral infections, such as flu (influenza), vary in severity, and no medication is useful in treating them. For certain kinds of influenza, *amantadine* has been effective in preventing onset. This drug is usually reserved for people at high risk. It has many side effects. The risk of complications from bacterial infections of the lungs after influenza is greater than with a cold. However, only if clear evidence indicates a complication are antibiotics necessary. Taking them to *prevent* complications can do more harm than good, because a more serious infection could result.

Should an older person receive an influenza vaccine?

This is a controversial matter. Each year the strain of flu virus changes, and the companies that make flu vaccines try to incorporate the most recent strains. If you are at special risk of a serious infection because of heart and lung disease, or if in the past you have had a prolonged illness with influenza, you should probably receive the vaccine. Since outbreaks usually occur in midwinter, the vaccine is given in the autumn so that your body has time to build up resistance. Many older people seem to benefit from the vaccines, and rarely do complications arise. A sore arm or a slight fever are usually the only side effects, and these are temporary.

How should an older person treat allergies that affect the upper respiratory system?

Some older people continue to suffer from allergic problems such as hay fever in their later years. However, in some the symptoms wane as they age, whereas others develop an allergy for the first time. The problem can be seasonal, either in the summer or winter, or it can occur throughout the year.

For many people a small dose of an antihistamine taken at night is sufficient to relieve the symptoms of a runny nose and coughing. However, antihistamines can cause drowsiness and should be taken only with your doctor's approval. Newer medications decrease allergic reactions if inhaled through the nose. These should not be confused with over-the-counter nasal sprays, which can be dangerous: They are often habit-forming and can cause a rise in blood pressure and a drying out of the nose. After a while they cease to work and may even aggravate your symptoms.

If a dripping nose or stuffiness is bothersome, see a specialist of the ear, nose, and throat. You could be suffering from an allergy to a substance that can be identified, and once it is removed, your symptoms may improve remarkably. Or, he may find another cause such as an infection or blockage that may require other treatment.

CHRONIC BRONCHITIS AND EMPHYSEMA

Chronic bronchitis is a condition in which the *bronchi* become inflamed and narrowed, thus interfering with the normal exchange of oxygen and carbon dioxide. It leads to shortness of breath, which often becomes progressively worse and eventually is incapacitating. Frequently, the breathlessness is accompanied by cough and the production of phlegm, and wheezing can occur during physical exertion or at rest.

Many people blame chronic bronchitis on gas poisoning (during the first world war), a fire, a bad bout of flu, automobile or air pollution, or an unhealthy work environment. However, the most important cause of this disease is cigarette smoking, which supplies a higher and more damaging amount of irritating substances to the lungs than any other source. It is usually heavy smokers who cite the other reasons, rather than admit that the damage is due to their own smoking habit, which injures the protective mechanism of the bronchi. Gradually, the lungs become more prone to infections and environmental pollution. What is called "smoker's cough" is really unrecognized chronic bronchitis.

Is chronic bronchitis curable?

The best cure is prevention. Once the changes in the bronchi have existed for a long time, the inflammation may continue even when you stop smoking. Parts of the lung that have already been seriously damaged cannot return to normal function. However, by kicking the smoking habit, you can prevent further damage and improve the natural defense of the lungs. In addition to not smoking, medications can help. Occasionally, antibiotics prevent repeated infections which could cause further lung damage.

Is physical activity good for chronic bronchitis?

In addition to good medical care, quitting smoking, and weight reduction, an exercise program supervised by a physician or therapist can improve lung function. Before starting the program, your physician will examine your heart and lungs, and *pulmonary function tests* may be done to measure improvements in your effort tolerance as the program proceeds.

An exercise plan should be gradual, with a slow progression in the type of activity and stress that is put on your heart and lungs. Many people who had been severely incapacitated have been brought to a level of function that allows them to carry out their normal everyday activities with reasonable comfort.

What medications are used to treat chronic bronchitis?

Bronchodilators reduce the spasmodic narrowing of the bronchi, which leads to wheezing. One type is *theophylline*, which can be given as a pill, a liquid, or, during serious attacks of wheezing, intravenously. Occasionally, it is given as a night suppository. Other drugs are those in the *adrenalin* group, although for the older person especially, adrenalin itself is rarely used. Its side effects can strain the heart by causing it to beat excessively fast and produce palpitations. Newer adrenalin-like medications in this group, available in pills and as an *inhaler*, dilate the bronchi without causing these cardiac side effects.

The inhaler is convenient and works rapidly. However, if you receive an inhaler and get no relief, tell your physician. Its use requires instruction and practice to learn how to activate the pressure device while inhaling. You must hold your breath for a few seconds to give the drug time to work before you exhale.

If you are severely incapacitated, *cortisone* medications might be needed. These are usually reserved for very ill patients or during life-threatening wheezing attacks. They have serious side effects, especially in the elderly, and long-term use should be avoided. Inhalers containing a cortisone-like medication have become available. They cause fewer side effects.

Antibiotics may be used during an acute flare-up of infection before serious complications occur. They are often given as soon as your phlegm becomes yellowish or green. However, sometimes bronchodilators alone will improve your symptoms.

If you already have chronic bronchitis, does it matter if you give up smoking?

Even though chronic bronchitis cannot be cured, there is an increased likelihood of infection so long as you continue to smoke. Some parts of the bronchi and lungs may still work adequately, and stopping smoking will allow these parts to remain unharmed. In addition, heavy smoking decreases the oxygen supply in the blood.

If you have been smoking for many years and have severe chronic bronchitis, you may think an occasional cigarette is acceptable. Although this is *not* good for your health, it is a reasonable compromise until you can stop altogether. Although pipe and cigar smoke is usually not inhaled, some smoke still reaches the bronchi and can cause damage. Remember, you are never too old to benefit from giving up tobacco.

What is the difference between chronic bronchitis and emphysema?

Emphysema causes the gradual breakdown of the thin walls that separate the alveoli (air sacs). The exchange of oxygen and carbon dioxide inside these enlarged alveoli (often called *bullae*) becomes inefficient. Chronic bronchitis and emphysema are commonly found together in people who are heavy cigarette smokers. This combination is called *chronic obstructive lung disease* or chronic lung disease. In those who suffer from emphysema alone, the bronchi are less affected than the lungs and the symptoms are somewhat different. There is usually less coughing, sputum production, and wheezing. However, breathlessness can be severe. Emphysema can occur in nonsmokers, but it is more common and more severe in those who smoke. If you suffer from emphysema alone without chronic bronchitis, bronchodilators and the adrenalin-like and cortisone-like drugs may be less effective.

UNUSUAL LUNG DISEASES

What unusual lung diseases occur in older people?

The most common lung diseases that occur in the older person are chronic bronchitis, emphysema, and pneumonia. The unusual diseases include infections caused by rare bacteria or viruses, as well as inflammation that can cause lung damage. Some inflammatory illnesses affect the lungs as well as other parts of the body and cause shortness of breath and cough.

How is lung disease diagnosed?

Pulmonary function tests are used to measure the activity of the lungs. They include tests that measure the amount of oxygen and carbon dioxide and show if the amount of air inhaled is adequate and if it is exhaled at a proper rate. Sometimes special X-rays called *tomograms* are necessary to illuminate a shadow that may not be easily interpreted by a regular chest X-ray. Occasionally, a physician will look into the bronchi and lungs with a *bronchoscope*, which allows him to take a sample of the sputum and cells from the bronchi and lungs. With newer instruments a bronchoscopic *lung biopsy* may also be taken. This is especially valuable in diagnosing unusual infections and tumors. It is a simple procedure that is done with a local anesthetic and has virtually no danger.

On rare occasions, when it is not possible to make a diagnosis with a bronchoscopic lung biopsy, a *needle biopsy* or an *open lung biopsy* may be necessary. A small sample of lung is either aspirated through the needle or removed through a small incision in the chest wall and analyzed. These procedures have little danger regardless of age.

I am reminded of an 88-year-old woman, who, prior to catching the flu, was able to walk three miles a day and swim for an hour three times a week. Soon after the infection began, she had difficulty breathing. During hospitalization she became so breathless that she could not leave her bed. Her daughter was very apprehensive because the tests already performed, including a bronchoscopy, were inconclusive.

When asked for permission to do an open lung biopsy, the daughter's response was, "She's too sick for such a test, isn't she?" It soon became clear to her that without a diagnosis and a chance of treatment her mother would die. She finally agreed. The pathologist reported that an unusual infection was producing scar tissue in the lungs and plugging up the alveoli. The patient was given cortisone therapy, which sometimes stops scar tissue from forming. Within forty-eight hours she was feeling better, and two weeks later she was discharged from the hospital. A year after her illness, she was able to walk two miles a day, although at a slightly slower pace than before. Two years later, at the age of 90, she still vacations in Florida and is very active. Without the biopsy which allowed proper treatment to be given, she probably would have died.

RESPIRATORS

Sometimes the lungs become so damaged that they cannot effectively carry out respiration. Therefore, oxygen does not reach the body in sufficient quantities and carbon dioxide builds up in the blood. This can be the result of something sudden or the culmination of a prolonged illness. If oxygen is lacking for even a short time, the body cannot survive unless breathing is assisted.

A *respirator* (breathing machine) allows the proper exchange of carbon dioxide and oxygen. A tube is passed through the larynx into the trachea. The tube is attached to a machine that takes over the movement of the muscles that normally control respiration. Oxygen is forced into the lungs and carbon dioxide is removed. Medications that decrease the natural tendency to breathe while the machine is in operation may be necessary for short periods. These drugs temporarily paralyze all the muscles, including those for breathing.

If the illness is acute and likely will improve with treatment, there is a very good chance that the older patient can eventually be taken off the respirator and be allowed to breathe naturally. A respirator is usually used only for severe lung infections until antibiotics or other treatments begin to take effect. Sometimes after major surgery, older people have difficulty establishing their normal breathing pattern. The respirator gives the body and lungs a chance to rest and regain strength in the meantime.

It is very unusual for a person to require a respirator permanently in order to live. Some people with chronic and progressive lung disease may require a respirator in their home on an intermittent basis, but this, too, is rare.

CHAPTER 11

Gastrointestinal Disease

The gastrointestinal tract, also called the *digestive system*, is responsible for the intake of food and its digestion, assimilation, and elimination. It begins with the mouth, where food is chewed and then broken down by *enzymes*. The *esophagus* (gullet) propels this partially digested food into the *stomach*. A *sphincter* (valve) separates the esophagus from the stomach and prevents food and stomach juices from passing backward into the esophagus.

Food is acted upon by *stomach acid* and enzymes before entering the *duodenum*, the passageway from the stomach to the *jejenum* and the *ileum*, which together with the duodenum make up the *small intestine* (small bowel). In the small intestine the food particles are digested into their elementary components of *carbohydrate, fat,* and *amino acids* (from protein). The lining of the small intestine engulfs the minute particles of food and *absorbs* them into the bloodstream and then into the *liver*.

After the food is absorbed, the leftover substances, including the fiber (roughage), are carried in the intestinal fluid, which

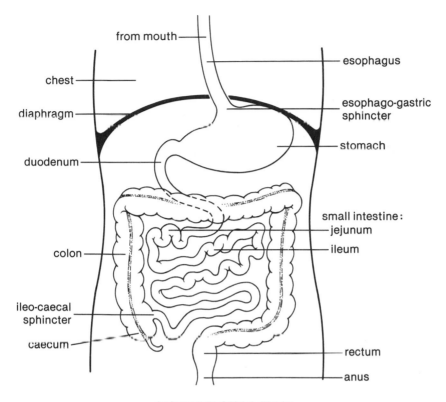

from mouth

esophagus

chest

esophago-gastric
sphincter

diaphragm

stomach

duodenum

small intestine:
jejunum

ileum

colon

ileo-caecal
sphincter

caecum

rectum

anus

GASTROINTESTINAL TRACT.

moves along the small bowel, and passes through another sphincter into the *caecum*. This is the first part of the *large intestine* (large bowel), which consists of the *colon* and *rectum*. In the colon water is absorbed by the body, and the water-free *feces* (stool, bowel movement) are then stored in the rectum. During a bowel movement the stool is expelled through the *anus*.

Several parts of the gastrointestinal system directly connected to the stomach and intestines are necessary for digestion. The *pancreas*, an organ that lies just behind the stomach, deep within the abdomen, produces *insulin*, which is necessary to metabolize sugar, and *pancreatic juice*, which contains enzymes. The pancreatic juice enters the duodenum through a small *pancreatic duct*.

The *biliary system* consists of the *liver, gallbladder*, and the biliary ducts, which connect them to the intestine. *Bile*, produced in the liver and stored in the gallbladder, passes into the duodenum and helps in the digestion and absorption of dietary fat. The liver, the factory of the body, receives the food that is absorbed through the intestine. The liver cells transform the nutrients into the building blocks of the body.

Many older people have gastrointestinal problems, but most illnesses can be diagnosed, and many respond well to treatment.

PEPTIC ULCERS

A peptic ulcer is one that is produced by the abnormal action of stomach (gastric) acid on the lining of the stomach or duodenum. A sore develops that gradually erodes the protective lining of the stomach or duodenum. Sometimes the ulcer penetrates the lining surface and enters the muscle layer.

Many factors lead to the production of ulcers in the older person. One factor is psychological makeup: Stress, anxiety, and tension often produce excess amounts of stomach acid, which can injure the cells lining the stomach. Also, medications such as antiinflammatory drugs (including aspirin) used to treat arthritis and rheumatism, and excess alcohol intake, can produce peptic ulcers.

What are the symptoms of a peptic ulcer?

The most common symptom is burning or gnawing abdominal pain. Stomach acid comes in contact with the ulcer because the protective lining has been injured. The pain is typically in the upper part of the abdomen, but it may go through to the back or to either side of the abdomen. It is often relieved by bland foods and antacids, but in some cases food makes the pain worse. Vomiting and gradual weight loss can occur. Sometimes the stools become black or dark red and have an offensive odor. This means that the ulcer is bleeding, and medical attention should be sought immediately.

In the older person ulcer pain may be less severe than in the younger person. Thus a physician will not always consider the possibility of an ulcer. Some older people deny any pain and may develop symptoms of an obstruction as the first symptom: Food will not pass from the stomach to the small bowel, which results in a bloated feeling and the regurgitation of food that was eaten many hours before. Some people develop complications without ever having experienced ulcer pain. Bleeding or perforation (piercing the wall) from an ulcer may be the first symptoms, and both are dangerous conditions.

What kind of peptic ulcers affect the elderly?

The two most common ulcers are the *duodenal ulcer* (duodenum) and the *gastric ulcer* (stomach). The duodenal ulcer, the more common type, is almost always benign. It causes pain, obstruction to the passage of food, perforation, or bleeding. The gastric ulcer, also often benign, likewise causes pain, perforation, or bleeding.

Do some ulcers become malignant?

In the older person especially, a gastric ulcer may be malignant and invade the rest of the stomach and spread to different parts of the body. In general, ulcers initially benign, duodenal or gastric, *remain* benign. Those ulcers diagnosed as malignant are usually so from the beginning. Years ago, when ulcer diagnosis depended primarily on X-rays, it was often impossible to determine whether an ulcer was benign or malignant. With newer techniques, however, physicians can make a diagnosis immediately.

Are ulcers more dangerous in the older person?

There is a higher incidence of malignant ulcers in the upper part of the stomach in older people. A biopsy will determine whether a gastric ulcer is benign or malignant. X-rays may be misleading. In the past antacid therapy was undertaken and the X-ray repeated to see if the ulcer had progressed. A biopsy done through a gastroscope is quicker and safer, however.

Older people are less tolerant of bleeding and perforations of an ulcer. When either occurs, treatment should be supervised by physicians and surgeons who have experience with older patients.

There is less room for procrastination when dealing with a bleeding ulcer as you grow older. The heart and circulation may not withstand the stress of the hemorrhage as well as a younger person's. If the bleeding continues (shown by black, sticky stools or by vomiting a dark coffeelike substance), emergency surgery may be necessary. Before surgery is decided upon, the physician will try to control the bleeding. A plastic tube inserted through the nose into the stomach draws up the acid and blood. If bleeding stops, the fluid loses its dark color. If it does not stop, despite acid-inhibiting medications, surgery may be necessary. The sooner the surgery is done, the better the chances for success.

How is a peptic ulcer diagnosed?

The most important clue to the diagnosis of peptic ulcers is the medical history. Once the diagnosis is suspected from the history, the usual procedure is to X-ray the stomach and duodenum with a *barium swallow* to determine the type of ulcer and its severity.

A direct look at the ulcer through a *gastroscope* may be helpful. During the examination photographs and biopsies of the ulcer can be taken. A biopsy that can be done through the gastroscope can help determine whether the ulcer is benign or malignant. The source and extent of bleeding can also be determined by this means. This can be useful because sometimes bleeding occurs from inflammation of the stomach (*gastritis*) or from ruptured veins or a tumor. The treatment of these conditions is different from ulcer therapy.

What is the best treatment for an ulcer?

Treatment begins by removing those factors that aggravate your ulcer tendency. This includes the withdrawal of drugs such as aspirin that increase acid secretion and decrease the defense mechanism of the stomach's lining. Alcohol should be avoided. In some people coffee and tea increase stomach acid production. Antacids taken in large quantities every one or two hours will decrease the effect of the stomach acid on the ulcer. There are many varieties with different amounts of active ingredients, so discuss the exact dosage with your physician. A large dose before bedtime is most important to help heal the ulcer and relieve the symptoms.

One new medication, *cimetidine*, prevents acid production by the stomach and helps improve the healing of ulcers. Because it is fairly new, it may be some time before its full benefit can be evaluated. Some older people experience a mild degree of mental confusion with this drug, in which case a decrease in dosage may be necessary.

This medication can be useful if you cannot tolerate frequent doses of antacids because of the taste or because they upset your bowel movements. It is sometimes used intravenously in urgent situations, as when an ulcer is bleeding or after ulcer surgery. Usually the pills are taken throughout the day and just prior to going to sleep. As the ulcer heals, the dosage is gradually decreased. However, in some people after the drug is discontinued, especially if done abruptly, new ulcers form. Therefore, the dosage is often decreased slowly before it is discontinued, and the person observed carefully for return of ulcer symptoms.

Is diet important in the treatment of peptic ulcers?

For many years diets played an essential role in the management of ulcers. Many people claimed to get relief by following a particular diet. Since most ulcers heal spontaneously or with the help of antacids, it is difficult to attribute it to one type of diet over another.

Some foods ease symptoms, whereas others aggravate them. You should eat small meals more frequently to keep acid production to a minimum. Food in the stomach also absorbs acid. Some physicians and patients feel that bland foods are helpful, others find that it is not so. Whatever diet you choose, make sure that it is well-balanced and comfortably tolerated. If you cannot find enough enjoyable foods, get advice from your physician or a dietitian.

Is surgery necessary for an ulcer?

With the newer medications the need for ulcer surgery has decreased. If you have unrelieved pain from an ulcer that has not responded to treatment with antacids or the newer medications (cimetidine), ulcer surgery should be considered. This is rarely the case in older people, however.

If your ulcer is bleeding, as shown by vomiting blood or passing black stools (digested blood within the stool), surgery may be necessary. If the bleeding is not profuse, medical management with antacids and acid inhibitors (cimetidine) is often tried first, especially if you have never taken these drugs in adequate amounts.

Occasionally, an ulcer penetrates the wall of the stomach and causes stomach juices to leak into the abdominal cavity. This is a life-threatening situation, and surgery to repair the damage is always essential.

There are various types of surgery for ulcer disease. The most common is a *vagotomy and pyloroplasty*. The *vagus nerve* controls the amount of acid produced by the stomach. By cutting it, less acid will be produced. However, this is not always successful. A pyloroplasty enlarges the opening from the stomach into the duodenum, thus allowing food to leave the stomach more quickly, which is often necessary when the vagus nerve is cut. Without the vagus nerve the stomach empties very slowly.

Sometimes a blockage prevents the propulsion of food from the stomach into the duodenum. This can occur if scar tissue from an ulcer has formed at the outlet of the stomach or duodenum. A *bypass* operation may be done, in which the stomach is attached to part of the jejunum so that food can enter the small intestine from the stomach for digestion.

In surgery for a perforation, the hole through which the stomach juice is leaking is closed. If necessary, the surgeon will perform a vagotomy and pyloroplasty at the same time in an attempt to prevent further ulcers from forming. This is not always possible if the surgery is urgent, so if a second operation is recommended, it may be worthwhile first to try to prevent further ulcers by taking antacids and acid inhibitors before agreeing to the operation. Also, discontinue medications such as aspirin or cortisone, which may have caused the perforation. If factors which caused the perforation are removed and ulcer medication taken, a second operation consisting of a vagotomy and pyloroplasty is rarely needed.

HIATUS HERNIA

The esophagus is separated from the stomach by the *diaphragm*, a muscle of the respiratory system that lies between the chest and the abdomen. At the junction of the esophagus and stomach is a valvelike mechanism (sphincter) that keeps the stomach contents (food and acid) from regurgitating into the esophagus. Sometimes part of the stomach may slide through the diaphragm and enter the chest. When this occurs, stomach juices pass into the esophagus and irritate it. The pouch of stomach that has been pushed into the chest is a *hiatus hernia*, and this can become twisted or bleed. It often exists without symptoms.

What are the symptoms of a hiatus hernia?

The most common symptoms are pain in the upper abdomen or lower chest and a sour or acid taste in the back of the mouth. This often occurs when you lie down or bend over. The feeling is often accompanied by heartburn or indigestion.

Some people develop a small degree of bleeding from the herniated (pouched) part of the stomach or from the lower part of the irritated esophagus. This bleeding may persist and eventually cause anemia. On occasion, the esophagus can become so inflamed and scarred that swallowing becomes difficult. Food can stick at the lower end of the esophagus and lead to severe vomiting following meals. In this case only fluids may be able to pass the narrowed junction between the esophagus and stomach.

Why are the symptoms of a hiatus hernia frequently confused with heart disease?

You may experience severe pain in the lower part of the chest because of stomach acid backing up into the esophagus. When this happens, the esophagus goes into spasm and can mimic the pain of a heart attack or angina pectoris. If you have experienced the pain of both angina pectoris and a hiatus hernia, you can usually tell them apart. However, many older people are inadvertently diagnosed as having angina pectoris

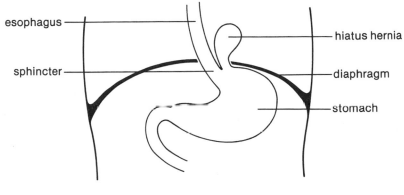

HIATUS HERNIA.

when, in fact, they have symptoms from a hiatus hernia, and vice versa.

One elderly lady, who was taking nitroglycerin tablets, nitroglycerin ointment, and beta-blockers for what she was told was severe angina pectoris, complained that her pain was still so severe that she could "hardly put on her shoes." The clue to the diagnosis was that the pain was bad when she bent over. Further tests ultimately showed that she had a large hiatus hernia. Treatment with antacids dramatically improved her so-called heart disease, and she was able to stop the medication for angina pectoris.

How is a hiatus hernia diagnosed?

If you have an *asymptomatic* hiatus hernia, a barium X-ray of your stomach may show some outpouching above the diaphragm. You will have few or no symptoms from this type of hiatus hernia and it can be shown that little gastric fluid is backing up from the stomach into the esophagus.

However, if you have the *symptoms* of a hiatus hernia, meaning a *symptomatic* hiatus hernia, the radiologist will try to demonstrate that the barium can flow backward from the

239

stomach into the esophagus. The X-ray may be inconclusive, however, and you may require a gastroscopy to confirm the diagnosis.

What is the best treatment for a hiatus hernia?

If you are obese, weight reduction may improve your symptoms by decreasing the amount of pressure in your abdomen. This causes less acid to back up from the stomach into the esophagus. Avoidance of tight garments such as girdles will also decrease acid regurgitation. If you are troubled with symptoms at night, you should raise the head of your bed on blocks to prevent stomach acid from reaching the esophagus.

The use of antacids to neutralize the irritating effects of stomach acid will usually decrease symptoms. With very severe attacks the use of an acid inhibitor, as in the treatment of peptic ulcers, may be effective.

New medications can improve the tone of the valve (sphincter) that separates the esophagus from the stomach, thus decreasing the amount of acid that can back up into the esophagus. The most important one is *metoclopramide*. Unfortunately, especially in the older person, this medication can lead to symptoms similar to Parkinson's disease. Sometimes a small amount, however, in addition to an antacid or acid inhibitor, will reduce the symptoms.

Is surgery ever necessary for a hiatus hernia?

With the newer drugs the need for surgery has greatly decreased. However, you may become so incapacitated by acid regurgitation, heartburn, pain, and bloating that you become fearful of eating and sleeping. In this case surgery can have dramatic effects. If an adequate trial of medical treatment is not effective, you should consider surgery. The risk is small compared to the major improvement that can result.

MALABSORPTION

The small bowel digests food with the assistance of *enzymes* produced by the pancreas and the small intestine. The enzymes allow the digested food to be absorbed by the intestine. It then goes to the liver, where it is metabolized and sent to the body.

If there is a decrease in the production of enzymes by the pancreas or the small intestine, digestion will be impaired, and the nutrients will not be absorbed. If the intestinal lining becomes diseased, food particles may not be able to pass into the bloodstream. These processes can cause malabsorption.

Malabsorption often leads to malnourishment because of the body's inability to break down the carbohydrates, fats, and proteins in the diet. You may lose excessive weight despite a normal or even increased appetite. You may experience a change in bowel habits with a tendency toward frequent, loose bowel movements. This is the result of undigested food passing through the intestines. Your stool may appear to be greasy and might float in the toilet bowl. The color is usually pale with a very strong odor.

If malabsorption continues over a long period, you might begin to suffer from anemia or other symptoms of vitamin deficiency, such as dry skin or a painful tongue. An accurate diagnosis should be made before these symptoms are treated.

What causes malabsorption?

Diseases of the pancreas can hinder or prevent the production of enzymes. You may have a history of inflammation of the pancreas *(pancreatitis)* or may have undergone previous abdominal surgery involving the pancreas. Sometimes the pancreas begins to slow down and cannot produce sufficient enzymes for proper digestion. Occasionally, tumors block the enzymes from reaching the intestine. The symptoms of malabsorption may be experienced before a tumor becomes evident.

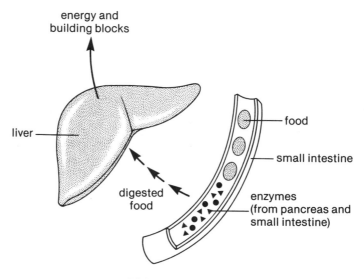

ABSORPTION OF FOOD

Individuals who have undergone surgery on their upper intestine may have had a bypass operation to relieve an obstruction, or part of the bowel may have been removed because of disease. This, too, can prevent proper and complete food absorption. Food passes through the intestine relatively quickly and exits from the body either undigested or only partially digested.

Previous bowel surgery might also lead to the formation of pouches in which bacteria grow and deplete some essential vitamins. Malabsorption of vitamin B_{12}, and subsequently anemia, can occur in this situation.

In an illness called *gluten enteropathy*, which is more commonly seen in younger people, the intestine becomes allergic to the gluten in flour. Eating ordinary bread and cereals causes the bowel to work poorly, and the result is malabsorption. An alteration in diet, as recommended by a physician or dietitian, will alleviate the symptoms. An accurate diagnosis cannot be made without special tests, perhaps including a biopsy of the

242

surface of the bowel to determine the exact cause of the malabsorptive process. This is done by swallowing a thin, plastic tube with a small device at its tip that removes a sample of bowel for microscopic examination. Also more common in younger individuals is *inflammatory bowel disease*, which may inhibit the proper absorption of food. It rarely starts during the later years, but may continue into them. The illness often causes abdominal pain and diarrhea, in addition to malabsorption.

How is malabsorption diagnosed?

Once you are suspected of suffering from malabsorption, your physician will look for evidence of pancreatic disease and intestinal disorders. Tests can determine whether enzymes are being produced in sufficient quantity for normal absorption. Blood tests measuring certain vitamins, minerals, and nutrients can help determine the degree to which absorption has been impaired. Your stool will be analyzed to see if it contains excessive fat, an important sign of malabsorption. X-rays, echograms, and nuclear scans of the pancreas will document disease, as will X-rays and a biopsy of the small intestine. Not all of these tests have to be done in every instance.

Is malabsorption treatable?

Depending on the underlying cause, most cases of malabsorption can be treated. A deficiency of pancreatic enzymes often improves with enzyme-replacement medication. If your symptoms subside with pancreatic enzyme replacement, there may be no need for additional tests unless other symptoms persist. In most cases you will regain your lost weight and notice an improvement in your bowel movements.

If you are allergic to the *gluten* in flour, a special diet will be prescribed. Sometimes vitamin supplements will be given if there is evidence that vitamin absorption is impaired.

THE LARGE BOWEL

The large bowel consists of the *colon, rectum,* and *anus.* During digestion, enzyme-rich fluid is mixed with and helps to digest the food as it passes through the small intestine. However, many undigested substances remain, including the fiber (roughage), which along with cells that come from the intestinal lining, make up the stool. In the colon, bacteria break down the substances in the stool, and the excess fluid is absorbed into the bloodstream. The stool gradually becomes solid and passes from the colon into the rectum, where it is stored.

The colon is surrounded by a layer of muscular cells that help propel the contents toward the rectum and anus. When the pressure within the abdomen increases and the muscle surrounding the rectum contracts, the bowel movement is pushed through the anus. A sphincter muscle prevents involuntary bowel movements.

Diseases of the large bowel can result from an impairment of its blood supply, abnormalities of the lining, or poor function of the muscular layer. Investigation of the bowel often requires an examination of the stool. Barium X-rays of the colon and a *sigmoidoscopy* or *colonoscopy* can be helpful in making the diagnosis.

ISCHEMIC BOWEL DISEASE

Ischemic bowel disease, due to a decreased blood supply to the bowel, can affect it in a number of ways. You may suffer weight loss due to malabsorption and experience abdominal pain (especially after meals) that is not relieved by antacids or other medications for indigestion.

The pain mechanism is similar to that of angina pectoris; hence, it is sometimes called *abdominal angina.* Very often, the diagnosis is elusive because it is difficult to differentiate this type of malabsorption from others, and there are also so many other causes of abdominal discomfort. Occasionally, the pain becomes severe and leads to a medical emergency. In this case, when the bowel's blood supply becomes dangerously low, an *angiogram* may show where the blood supply is impaired.

You can also develop bleeding from the bowel as a result of the decreased blood supply which can be painless, although often there is some abdominal discomfort during an attack. This can be a very frightening experience, and it frequently leads to hospitalization. The bleeding usually stops by itself, but it may recur. Sometimes after bleeding, there may be some damage and scarring of the bowel, which can lead to partial or complete blockage. This is rare, but when it occurs, surgery to relieve the obstruction is sometimes required, if the blockage is severe.

What is the treatment for a poor blood supply to the bowel?

In most instances there is no specific treatment. Because a number of arteries are often involved, it is usually not possible to replace them with artificial blood vessels. If the aorta (the main artery of the body) is involved, a surgeon may recommend a synthetic aortic graft.

If a blood vessel to the bowel becomes completely blocked, the bowel will become severely damaged and eventually die. Immediate surgical removal is crucial. This potentially life-saving surgery can be accomplished successfully, however. If a large part of the bowel has to be removed, malabsorption may occur, so special diets will be recommended to assure adequate nutrition.

DIVERTICULAR BOWEL DISEASE

The lining of the large bowel has many smooth undulations that increase the surface area that absorbs liquid. The lining is surrounded by a muscular layer that helps propel the feces through the colon to the rectum and then through the anus.

245

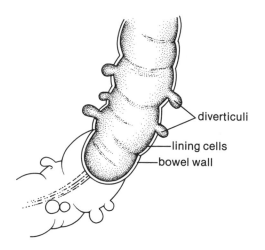

diverticuli

lining cells

bowel wall

DIVERTICULAR BOWEL DISEASE.

Many older people have a great many "outpouchings" of the bowel's lining that protrude through the muscular layer. The little pouches are called *diverticulum*, and the condition is referred to as *diverticulosis*. In most people the pouches are discovered during a barium enema that is being done for another reason. Usually, there are no symptoms. When the pouches become inflamed, *diverticulitis* results.

The exact cause of diverticulosis is not known, but some evidence suggests that it occurs in people who also suffer from chronic constipation. Perhaps excessive pressure within the colon causes the lining to protrude. Some people feel that a diet that is very low in fiber may contribute to the disease.

What are the symptoms of diverticular bowel disease?

In most people diverticular bowel disease consists only of diverticulosis and causes very few problems. In some, however, a diverticulum can bleed painlessly and cause blood to be passed through the anus. Occasionally, diverticuli become acutely inflamed and cause a blockage of the bowel. Pain, fever, and tenderness can occur when many diverticuli become inflamed or infected. A diverticulum can rupture and cause *peritonitis*, a severe abdominal infection. It can also "stick" to organs such as the bladder and cause them to become inflamed.

What is the treatment?

When the condition does not cause symptoms, only a high-fiber diet is necessary, although stool softeners and medications that increase its bulk, such as *psyllium mucilloid*, are often useful as well. During an attack of diverticulitis the treatment often temporarily requires a totally fluid diet. Sometimes intravenous feeding may be necessary to allow the bowel to rest for a few days. Antispasmodics, antibiotics, and painkillers can decrease spasm and inflammation and eradicate infection. If a blockage occurs, or if one of the pouches perforates and the infection spreads to the abdomen, surgery will be necessary. These complications are rare.

How can diverticular disease be prevented?

All the factors causing diverticular bowel disease are not known. Many older people have in the past been warned against eating fresh fruits, vegetables, and whole-grain breads and cereals. Unfortunately, this appears to be erroneous. If anything, a fiber-poor diet aggravates the condition.

If a diagnosis of diverticular disease is made, you should gradually increase your intake of fiber. Although this will not cure the disease, it may improve your symptoms.

FUNCTIONAL BOWEL DISORDERS

Functional usually means of a nonphysical nature. Many older people often have multiple abdominal complaints. But many of these, in fact, are not the result of any discoverable disease within the gastrointestinal tract. In general, the prognosis is good. However, patients often have many tests before the physician realizes that the symptoms are caused by factors other than serious bowel disease.

What are the
symptoms of functional bowel disease?

Unfortunately, the same type of symptoms that occur in other kinds of abdominal diseases also occur in functional bowel disease. The common complaints are indigestion, belching, nausea, vomiting, diarrhea, and constipation. Loss of appetite and various types of abdominal pain also occur.

Often your physician will find nothing in your abdomen or bowel to explain your symptoms. Tests including X-rays, nuclear scans, and echograms may be done but no explanation found. Medications that are usually successful in other types of abdominal disease may have poor results. Your physician becomes puzzled and frustrated, and you become unduly fearful as your discomfort persists.

Why is this disease so common in older people?

In many instances functional bowel disease is a reflection of emotional problems, perhaps because of the loss of loved ones or a feeling of isolation and uselessness. Some people become fearful of death and develop "cancerphobia." They may even begin to develop symptoms that support their fears.

Sometimes the bowel complaints are a result of depression. In the older person this should not be overlooked. Once an adequate investigation has been completed and your physician can assure you emphatically that you do not suffer from cancer or some other serious bowel disease, you should examine the emotional and social aspects of your life with him.

Some people improve with psychotherapy, antidepressants, stool softeners, and a simplified diet containing more fiber.

There may be a place for the occasional use of tranquilizers and antispasmodic medications. Sometimes the symptoms cannot be completely relieved, and you should try to direct attention away from your bowel and your diet and focus on more productive aspects of your life.

BOWEL TUMORS

As one grows older, the incidence of tumors of the large bowel increases. The cause is uncertain, although they run in some families. It is not clear whether diet plays an important role. Both benign and malignant tumors occur in the bowel and may cause similar symptoms.

What are the symptoms of a bowel tumor?

Occasionally, tumors of the lower bowel are discovered during a rectal examination or *sigmoidoscopy*, which is frequently done as part of a periodic checkup. X-rays of the bowel done for other reasons may also show a tumor.

Many bowel tumors first show themselves by bleeding. You may actually see the red blood during or after a bowel movement. Often the amount is so small as to be unnoticeable. This is known as *occult bleeding*, and it often shows itself through anemia. To determine its presence, the stool is chemically tested for evidence of blood. Bleeding from the bowel, or anemia combined with the finding of blood in the stool, should lead to a full investigation of the intestinal tract.

A bowel tumor may cause a change in your bowel habits, producing either constipation or diarrhea. Occasionally, they alternate. In such cases an intestinal examination is mandatory.

How is the diagnosis made?

If there is a suspicion of a bowel tumor, the usual procedure is to do a rectal examination and check the stool for occult blood. A *sigmoidoscopy* to observe the lower bowel is usually done after the rectal examination. If the tumor appears, a biopsy can determine if it is benign or malignant. A barium enema is often the next test. If this does not reveal the tumor, your stomach and upper intestines may be X-rayed. It is less common for tumors to be found in the upper intestines, although tumors of the stomach, both benign and malignant, do occur.

The relatively new procedure known as *colonoscopy* has become helpful in diagnosing tumors of the lower bowel. A colonoscope, a long, flexible device, is inserted through the anus and passed along the full length of the bowel. If a tumor is seen, it can be biopsied through the instrument. Some benign tumors can be removed through the colonoscope, depending on their size and location, which means surgery can be avoided.

Sometimes an *angiogram* is necessary, especially if there is profuse bleeding from the tumor at the time of the examination.

Is surgical removal of a tumor dangerous?

The risk of having surgery must always be weighed against the risk of the disease. Bowel tumors are serious whether benign or malignant. The danger of surgery is relatively small compared to the hazardous effects of a tumor. With modern surgical techniques most older people can be brought through major large-bowel surgery with relatively little risk.

If a malignant tumor is found, is surgery necessary?

Many people and some physicians assume that if a bowel tumor is malignant the outlook is very poor. Some even feel that surgery will only increase the amount of suffering. In the vast majority of cases this is not so.

Surgery is recommended for a number of reasons. If found and treated early, some large bowel malignant tumors can be cured. A malignant tumor should be removed in order to prevent potential bowel obstruction, a dangerous situation that may require emergency surgery. Removing the malignant tumor before obstruction may not always cure the long-term effects of the tumor, but it will often prevent a blockage of the bowel.

Frequently, one can expect a good result from surgical removal of a malignant tumor. X-rays and nuclear scans are often done before surgery to see if the tumor has spread to other parts of the body. With newer surgical techniques the tumor may be removed and the bowel resewn in a way that will allow normal function.

Sometimes a *colostomy* may be required either temporarily or permanently. This allows the bowel movement to leave the body through an opening on the abdominal wall. A plastic bag catches the stool for disposal. In some cases the colostomy may be closed at a later date and bowel function returned to normal.

Radiation or chemotherapy may be required after surgery to improve the results of treatment. In some cases radiation to the rectum has been used with success to shrink a malignant tumor and prevent obstruction and spread. This type of therapy should be discussed with your physician. Quite often something positive can be done to decrease the likelihood of bowel obstruction at the time a tumor is first discovered.

The effects of a malignant tumor can return at a later date. Although the drugs available are not completely effective, various forms of chemotherapy are being improved.

BLEEDING IN THE GASTROINTESTINAL TRACT

Bleeding in the gastrointestinal tract, which can occur from the esophagus to the anus, must always be taken seriously. Depending on the area of bleeding, the symptoms can vary.

Bleeding in the esophagus or stomach, if profuse, may reveal itself by being vomited as bright red blood. This, of course, can be frightening. It sometimes occurs in people who have severe liver disease, peptic ulcers, stomach tumors, or inflammation of the esophagus. If the blood is not immediately vomited, it is converted by the stomach acid into a gritty brown material similar to *coffee grounds*. In fact, medical people refer to it by this name. This may be vomited or passed into the intestinal tract, where it exits through the anus as a black, sticky material called *melena*.

Less profuse bleeding from the esophagus or stomach, as may occur in a hiatus hernia or peptic ulcer, may not be noticed in the bowel movement. The stool will appear normal in color, and it will not have the offensive odor that is associated with melena. This is *occult bleeding* and the usual symptom is anemia.

Bleeding from the small intestine, which is rarely profuse and quite uncommon, usually causes occult bleeding and anemia. Large-bowel blood loss may be the result of tumors, inflammation, or ischemic bowel disorders. There may be no other symptoms of the many diseases that cause large-bowel blood loss other than the bleeding itself. Often it is discovered because a person becomes weak from anemia. Although the anemia itself can be treated with iron pills, tests should be done to determine the cause of the bleeding. In many cases an illness will be discovered for which there is successful treatment.

If you develop anemia and blood is found in your stool, you should expect a thorough investigation, which may include a rectal examination and a *sigmoidoscopy*, followed by a *barium enema* and perhaps a *colonoscopy*. If these procedures do not reveal the source of bleeding, an upper gastrointestinal series (G.I. series) and perhaps a *gastroscopy* will be required. In exceptional circumstances, if bleeding is rapid and profuse, an *angiogram* of the abdominal blood vessels may be necessary. If blood is being vomited, a plastic tube is inserted through the nose into the stomach to measure the degree of bleeding and suck out the stomach acid, which is mixed with blood. This is helpful in decreasing the degree of hemorrhage.

In almost every case a source of bleeding can be found. Even if you see blood in your stool only once in a while, report it to your physician at once before more severe symptoms develop.

HEMORRHOIDS

Hemorrhoids are the result of a protrusion of veins through the anus, caused particularly by straining during a bowel movement. They are often found in people who suffer from chronic constipation and whose diet is low in fiber. Eventually the bulging veins protrude through the anus even when there is no straining.

The symptoms vary according to the severity of the hemorrhoids. There may be a feeling of fullness at the anus, which may become exaggerated during and after a bowel movement. Quite frequently, a small amount of bleeding may be noticed during or after a bowel movement. The blood may be seen on the stool itself, in the toilet, or on the toilet paper. However, the bleeding is usually not severe enough to cause anemia. Occasionally, a hemorrhoidal vein becomes trapped outside the anus and a blood clot forms within it. This can cause excruciating pain and swelling that can make walking or sitting impossible until treatment is received.

If you have never experienced hemorrhoids, another underlying cause in addition to excessive straining at stool should be looked for. Sometimes a tumor of the bowel can cause excessive pressure on the veins in the anus and show itself as hemorrhoids for the first time in later life. If you are anemic and have bleeding hemorrhoids, your bowel should be investigated. If it is assumed that the anemia is caused by bleeding from the hemorrhoids alone, a more serious condition such as bowel cancer may accidentally be overlooked.

What is the best treatment for hemorrhoids?

For most people hemorrhoids are more of an inconvenience than a danger. They usually can not only be treated but also prevented. Your diet should include enough roughage (fiber) to prevent you from having to strain during a bowel movement. In addition, you may do very well with stool softeners, occasional mineral oil, and increased liquids.

Local treatment with anesthetic and cortisone ointments or suppositories is sometimes necessary during an episode of severe pain or when a blood clot forms within a hemorrhoid. Sometimes a quick, simple incision and removal of the blood clot may lead to immediate relief of the pain. This can usually be done in the doctor's office. Sitting in a warm bath or applying warm compresses can be very soothing.

It is unusual for an older person to require surgery for the relief of hemorrhoidal symptoms. Preventive measures and local therapy should be tried before surgery is considered.

Recent advances in minor surgery have been made that can greatly relieve the discomfort from very troublesome hemorrhoids. These techniques include tying off the engorged blood vessels under a local anesthetic or with no anesthetic at all. It can often be done in the office of a well-trained surgeon specializing in this type of treatment. Sometimes freezing of the hemorrhoids is done in conjunction with the tying, and this may remove the hemorrhoid more effectively. No one should have to suffer repeatedly from the discomfort of hemorrhoids. Simple, good, and effective treatment is available regardless of age.

PANCREATIC DISEASE

The pancreas lies deep within the abdomen behind the stomach. One group of pancreatic cells produces the hormone *insulin*, which is necessary for the normal control and utilization of sugar. Other cells produce the pancreatic juice, which contains *enzymes* necessary for the digestion of food. Disease of the pancreas can result in a decrease in the production of insulin and enzymes. When there is too little insulin, diabetes mellitus occurs. A decrease in the production of enzymes can result in malabsorption. Inflammation of the pancreas can occur in people who drink too much alcohol or have gallbladder disease. Tumors can develop in the pancreas and can be either benign or malignant. Because the pancreas is seated so deeply within the abdomen, diagnosis may be difficult, but X-rays of the stomach and duodenum and newer procedures, including the abdominal echogram and CAT scan, have been instrumental in elucidating problems and have decreased the need for angiograms, which in the past were frequently required for diagnosis.

Blood tests are also useful to examine whether the enzymes are working properly. During an attack of *pancreatitis* (inflammation of the pancreas), excess enzymes will be found in the blood. The results of pancreatic enzyme deficiency may be seen in blood tests that demonstrate malabsorption.

Sometimes it is necessary to take a biopsy of the pancreas. This can now be done without surgery by inserting a thin needle into the pancreas with the assistance of an echogram. The procedure has little danger and may allow a diagnosis of pancreatic disease to be made in some instances without abdominal surgery.

What is pancreatitis?

Pancreatitis is an inflammation of the pancreas in which the enzymes escape into the abdominal cavity. The enzymes act on the abdominal tissues and cause fluid and sometimes blood to leak into the abdomen. It is a serious condition when it occurs suddenly, and it often leads to severe abdominal pain and sometimes shock.

The most common cause of acute pancreatitis in the older population is the passage of a gallstone through the biliary duct, which is connected to the pancreatic duct. The pain begins like that of *biliary colic*, but it becomes more severe and persistent and may affect the whole abdomen, making it impossible for you to find a comfortable position. Pancreatitis can also occur after many years of alcohol abuse. Attacks may come and go, each one leaving its toll of damage on the pancreas. This is called *chronic pancreatitis*.

In most cases, other than when alcohol abuse is likely,

pancreatitis is caused by gallbladder disease. It is usually necessary to put the digestive system at complete rest by inserting a thin plastic tube into the stomach through the nose to remove the digestive juices. Fluids are given intravenously. Usually a strong pain medication is necessary, and sometimes antibiotics are given to prevent infection. Surgery, however, is rare, and it is usually not successful.

After the attack has subsided gallbladder X-rays will be taken. If the gallbladder is diseased, surgery to remove it is usually recommended, rather than running the risk of another attack of pancreatitis. Sometimes after an attack of pancreatitis, an inflammatory *cyst* (collection of fluid) forms. This can cause abdominal pain and pressure and may require surgical drainage of the fluid in order to alleviate the symptoms.

Are pancreatic tumors dangerous?

Because the pancreas sits so deeply within the abdomen, it is often difficult to diagnose tumors when they are small. Benign tumors of the pancreas are much less common than malignant ones. One type of benign tumor produces excess amounts of insulin and therefore causes low blood sugar *(hypoglycemia)*. The symptoms are sweating and fainting, and, in the older person, mental confusion. The effect is similar to an insulin overdose. The symptoms are eradicated once the tumor is removed. Other benign tumors are even less prevalent and may cause unusual symptoms (such as diarrhea) that do not respond to usual treatment.

The most common type of pancreatic tumor, *carcinoma of the pancreas (pancreatic cancer)*, usually has an insidious onset with vague abdominal symptoms. Weight loss, bloating, and abdominal discomfort are often experienced. Quite frequently, the individual may become depressed and undergo psychological treatment before the malignancy reveals itself. Investigations to show the tumor are not always successful,

especially in the early stages, and treatment is usually unsatisfactory.

GALLBLADDER DISEASE

The gallbladder is a small sack that lies just under the liver in the upper right-hand side of the abdomen. It is connected to the liver by *hepatic ducts,* which channel the *bile* produced by the liver into the gallbladder for storage between meals. Bile aids in digestion by breaking up dietary fats. The *bile duct* connects the gallbladder to the duodenum and conducts the flow of bile during meals.

Approximately 10 percent of all adults have *gallstones.* In middle-aged adults the percentage rises to 20, and in people over 65 gallstones can be detected in about 30 percent. As a consequence, gallbladder surgery is one of the most commonly performed operations today.

The cause of gallstone formation is complex and only partially understood. It is known that some people have a hereditary tendency to develop gallstones, and people who are obese are at an increased risk. Some evidence suggests that a high-calorie, high-carbohydrate diet also augments the likelihood of gallstone formation, and some researchers claim that a low-fiber diet increases the chance of gallstones.

Most gallbladder disease is associated with gallstones. A great deal of work has gone into trying to discover what other factors are responsible. It seems that some people produce bile that has an imbalance between the normal amount of *cholesterol* and *bile salts,* which normally dissolve cholesterol. If the imbalance persists for a long period, the cholesterol gradually settles out of the bile and collects as gallstones. These gradually grow and begin to damage the gallbladder by pressure, by facilitating infection, or by blocking the bile ducts.

Most people are unaware that they have gallstones, and sometimes they are discovered during an X-ray done for

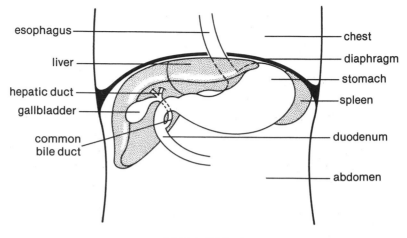

esophagus — — chest

liver — — diaphragm

— stomach

hepatic duct — — spleen

gallbladder —

common bile duct — — duodenum

— abdomen

BILIARY SYSTEM.

another purpose. If a gallbladder X-ray shows gallstones, this does not necessarily mean that they are the cause of your abdominal discomfort.

Since the formation of gallstones usually starts during your younger years, there is probably little that you can do later on to prevent their appearance. In most instances the stones may already have absorbed calcium, which increases their hardness. If you know that your family tends to develop gallstones, you should try to keep your weight down, avoid a high-fat diet, and increase the fiber in your diet. However, if the stones have already formed, these steps may not have any positive effect.

What problems are caused by gallstones?

A number of conditions are caused by gallstones. One is inflammation and infection of the gallbladder, known as *acute cholecystitis*. You may experience pain in the upper right side of your abdomen, along with fever, chills, nausea, and vomiting. This is a serious illness that usually requires hospitalization.

Sometimes an abscess of the gallbladder occurs if antibiotic treatment is delayed or proves to be ineffective.

In *biliary colic* a small stone is passed through the bile duct and causes spasm, which results in severe abdominal pain. In many cases the gallstone is either passed into the intestine or returns to the gallbladder and the symptoms subside. If the gallstone blocks the bile duct, however, you may develop jaundice as a result of bile accumulating in the body. The liver eventually can be severely damaged unless the obstruction is relieved.

During the passage of a gallstone, the pancreas, whose duct shares a common entrance to the duodenum with the gallbladder, may become inflamed, resulting in *pancreatitis*, with abdominal pain, fever, and shock. This condition can be life threatening and requires urgent hospitalization.

You may have repeated attacks of fever, chills, and a blood and liver infection as the result of a partial blockage of the bile ducts from gallstones. This condition, known as *cholangitis*, can lead to severe infections as well as shock.

When is gallbladder surgery necessary?

Finding gallstones on a routine X-ray is not in itself a reason to have your gallbladder removed. If you have vague, nonspecific abdominal symptoms, the discovery of gallstones does not necessarily mean that they are causing your symptoms. In fact, in many cases the removal of the gallbladder for these complaints is very disappointing because the symptoms may persist.

A blockage of the bile duct from a gallstone usually requires surgery, but some new methods allow a blocked bile duct to be relieved through a modified *gastroscopy* without surgery. This is not available everywhere, however, but eventually it will be used more frequently for the elderly when surgery may be too risky. I recommend gallbladder surgery only after an acute gallbladder episode, such as cholecystitis, billiary colic, cholangitis, or pancreatitis. The infection or blockage will first be treated medically with intravenous fluids and antibiotics until surgery can be done safely.

Whenever possible, the operation should be done on an elective basis, and not as an emergency. If you have diabetes mellitus, you are at greater risk of complications of gallstones, so earlier surgery might be considered.

Can gallstones be treated without surgery?

A low-fat diet is sometimes helpful in decreasing the number of biliary colic attacks, although it does nothing to dissolve the gallstones. Several drugs that can dissolve *cholesterol* gallstones, which are found mostly in younger people, are being studied. Their effect is temporary, and when stopped the stones may return.

In the future it may be possible to treat gallstones without surgery. Presently, however, surgery is necessary.

LIVER DISEASE

The liver, which makes the building blocks required for growth and maintenance of health, metabolizes proteins, carbohydrates, and fats and breaks down the body's waste products. Your liver can be damaged either by illness, medications, or alcohol. Injury to the liver often shows itself by the accumulation of *bile* in the body, which leads to *jaundice*, a yellow discoloration of the skin and eyes. The greater the degree of jaundice, the more severe the liver disease.

It may take many years before the effects of liver damage appear. Unfortunately, once severely injured, either acutely or chronically, it may no longer work effectively. The acute causes of liver disease may improve with treatment, whereas the long-standing causes usually do not.

Is alcohol dangerous to the liver?

There is no question that alcohol causes serious liver damage. The injury is directly proportional to the amount of alcohol used and the frequency and duration with which it is taken. The long-term effect of heavy alcohol abuse causes *cirrhosis of the liver,* a disease in which the liver cells gradually become replaced by scar tissue, which creates pressure on the blood vessels in the abdomen. The liver can no longer build proteins and get rid of waste products. Susceptibility to infection increases, and jaundice may result from the accumulation of waste products. Fluid often gathers within the abdomen and legs because the blood vessels cannot drain effectively through the scarred liver.

One serious complication caused by alcoholic liver disease is bleeding from the esophagus. The veins that cannot drain through the liver find a pathway through the esophagus. When the veins burst, severe, dangerous bleeding results. The best treatment is to stop drinking and seek help from your physician and from a group such as Alcoholics Anonymous. Once the disease is permanently established, medications may temporarily improve symptoms and decrease fluid accumulation. However, there may continue to be a gradual deterioration in health that gives rise to serious complications.

Can the liver be damaged by medication?

Many medications pass through the liver and are metabolized. Some medications, if taken too frequently, can cause liver damage. Some tranquilizers *(phenothiazines)* and medications used for anesthesia can occasionally cause an inflammation of the liver, but this will disappear when the medication is stopped. The inflammation occurs infrequently, but it should be considered by your physician if your liver becomes damaged while you are taking medications or after your have had surgery.

What other diseases can affect the liver?

Although more prevalent in younger people, *viral hepatitis* may occur. This infection can cause severe jaundice, but in most instances it improves with time and recovery will be good.

Older people with gallbladder disease may develop liver problems. A blockage of the bile duct can cause a backup of bile and a swelling of the liver. Infections from the gallbladder may spread to the liver, causing inflammation or infection. This is usually treated along with the gallbladder disease, however. Rarely, an abscess forms within the liver, and it must be treated surgically and with high doses of antibiotics. If found and treated early, the results are usually good.

A common disease affecting the liver of older people is cancer. Although a tumor may begin its growth in the liver, especially in alcoholic liver disease, most liver tumors have spread from other parts of the body or from the gastrointestinal tract.

If a tumor has been found in your stomach, bowel, or pancreas, your liver may already have been affected, although this is often not the case. The liver may become invaded a long time after the first symptoms and treatment of the original tumor has occurred. And possibly the liver may never be damaged by malignant growths from other parts of the body.

Malignancies affecting the liver are usually difficult to treat. By the time a liver malignancy is found, the disease is well advanced. The main direction of treatment is to ensure comfort with medications. Although the progress of the illness may be rapid, in some older individuals it can be very slow and without a great deal of discomfort.

DIET AND THE GASTROINTESTINAL TRACT

A number of gastrointestinal conditions require changes in diet. Whatever else the diet contains, it should be well balanced and have a caloric content that avoids obesity. If you suffer from ulcer disease or a hiatus hernia, you may find that certain foods aggravate your symptoms. Caffeine, alcohol, and certain spices seem to intensify the symptoms in some people, whereas others appear to tolerate them quite well. It is usually recommended that meals be small and taken more often than three times a day. You may feel better if your food is relatively bland, but this may be more psychological than real. Many people enjoy all foods quite comfortably and only have to modify their diets when they have symptoms. If you have gallbladder disease, you may feel better when you reduce your fat intake. If you are bothered by eggs and greasy foods, avoid them.

You may experience gas, bloating, and diarrhea if you have lactose intolerence caused by a deficiency in the enzyme *lactase*. Avoiding milk products may relieve the symptoms. A new product containing *lactase* is available that can be added to milk products and replace the missing enzyme needed to digest lactose.

An increase in fiber through whole-grain cereals and breads, fruits, and vegetables is recommended. This is especially good if you suffer from chronic constipation, hemorrhoids, and diverticular bowel disease. If you have lost your taste for these foods, you should begin with small quantities. A fair program would be to try each new fruit or vegetable separately to see if it agrees with you.

CHAPTER 12

Infections

As people get older, they become more susceptible to infection because the normal defense mechanisms begin to deteriorate. There is not only an increased risk of acquiring an infection, but the illness itself may last longer and respond less quickly to treatment. The signs of infection in older individuals are less vivid than in younger people.

The most serious infections are usually caused by *bacteria*. They either invade the body from outside or live within it without causing harm until the defenses fail. Another common cause of infection is a *virus*. This usually causes less severe infections, such as colds and influenza. For the most part, unless you have some other serious disease, you will overcome virus illnesses by yourself. However, more threatening virus infections occasionally afflict older people.

It is important to differentiate between bacterial and virus infections because the treatments are quite different. At present, there is no effective cure for virus infections; antibiotics have no effect at all. Although many people receive antibiotics for virus infections, the illness improves by itself, and not because of the antibiotic. However, bacterial infections may progress and cause serious, often life-threatening illnesses if they are not treated with antibiotics.

One of the problems of diagnosing infections in older people is that many of the usual symptoms may be lacking. *Fever* is one of the important signs of infection, and in younger people it is unlikely that an infection is present if there is no fever. As you grow older however, your fever control mechanism does not work as efficiently, so the lack of fever does not mean that you do not have an infection. Sometimes the opposite occurs. During an infection your fever may become extremely elevated and you may perspire excessively. You may experience serious effects from the fever alone, especially if you are unable to drink enough fluids to meet your body's needs. In this circumstance the fever may be not only an important symptom of an infectious illness, but it may cause its own problems, which have to be treated by replacing the lost fluids.

At other times a fever occurs that is not caused by an infection. Sometimes multiple treatments with antibiotics are tried with no effect before it becomes apparent that the illness is not the result of an infection.

PNEUMONIA

One frequent illness that affects older individuals is pneumonia, an infection of the lungs. The respiratory system and lungs have a protective mechanism that usually clears out unwanted bacteria and viruses, but when the protection breaks down, bacteria or viruses may grow and pneumonia results.

It is often said that pneumonia is a friend of the aged. This means that during the later stages of life or following a serious illness, pneumonia may be the illness that finally results in death. However, pneumonia can occur even when your health is good. A progression of the infection or death would not only be unexpected, but would indeed be unwelcome.

Today, pneumonia is far less dangerous than it used to be. I have seen many very elderly people who developed severe lung infections and became extremely ill to the point that the families and even some medical staff thought they had no chance of recovery. But often the patient was returned to a very satisfactory level of health and activity.

Do certain circumstances make you susceptible?

After flulike illnesses or other viral infections that may weaken the lungs' normal defenses, pneumonia may set in. Physicians frequently see older people who have suffered from flu for a few days and then develop chest pain, a cough that produces *purulent* (yellowish-green) phlegm, and fever. Confusion, dehydration, and emotional agitation commonly occur. Pneumonia can occur after surgery that required an anesthetic and result in a clouded mental state, as well as cough and fever. Because of postoperative pneumonia, surgery is a potential danger in the older person.

Some older people have neurological problems such as strokes or similar diseases that interfere with normal swallowing and coughing. The usually protective cough reflex is lost, and they may repeatedly inhale infected material into their lungs, where the bacteria multiply. This is called *aspiration (inhaled) pneumonia*, and it is common in weakened older people.

In all cases pneumonia may be devastating if left untreated. The lung infection progresses and interferes with the exchange of oxygen and carbon dioxide, leading to serious effects on the whole body. Bacteria may enter the bloodstream and cause further infections throughout the body. The high fever causes loss of fluids and leads to dehydration, which can exaggerate the effects of the pneumonia. Frequently, mental confusion occurs, which may result in inappropriate behavior and be potentially dangerous. One may wander, fall, and cause bodily injury. Rapid diagnosis and treatment is often very successful in reversing the illness.

Can pneumonia be prevented?

Many causes of pneumonia are difficult to avoid. It is possible, however, to reduce the risk and improve your chance of recovery.

Heavy smokers have a much greater chance of experiencing a lung infection because the natural defense mechanism is compromised by the constant irritation of cigarette smoke. Your nutritional health may play a role in preventing pneumonia. Obesity decreases the proper movement of the lungs. This is more serious if you are about to have an operation, especially an abdominal one. After surgery it is important to be able to take deep breaths and cough if you are to avoid a lung infection.

In many older people pneumonia follows a cold or influenza. There is no special cure for these viral illnesses, although vaccines may prevent certain influenza infections. Flu shots are usually available in the early fall, and they seem to be effective.

Recently, a vaccine has been developed that may prevent the occurrence of bacterial pneumonia caused by the *pneumococcus* bacterium. This variety can be very serious in the older person. Although the pneumococcus is responsible for many lung infections, it is not the cause of all of them, so the benefits of the vaccine have not been completely determined. However, many physicians do give it to their older patients in addition to a flu shot.

If you have serious diseases of the heart and lungs, you might benefit from these vaccines. Although not completely foolproof, they are probably useful. However, they should not be used instead of the other general good health measures, such as cessation of cigarette smoking and weight loss, but in addition to them.

What can be done when pneumonia is suspected?

When pneumonia is caused by bacteria, antibiotic treatment is mandatory. You may require hospitalization if the infection is advanced. In many instances, during the early stages, antibiotic therapy given at home may be adequate if you can be examined often by a nurse or physician. It is very important to drink lots of fluids because dehydration can be dangerous. If adequate fluids cannot be taken by mouth, intravenous therapy is often required. For this, hospital care is usually needed.

It is sometimes difficult for the family of an older person to understand why so much effort is going into treating their aged parent suffering from pneumonia. Some of the procedures may appear cruel. Frequently, it is necessary to take a sample of phlegm, and if you are confused and dehydrated, you may not be able to give it by yourself. The physician will draw out the sputum through a plastic tube, which can cause momentary discomfort. This allows him to choose the right antibiotic.

Blood tests are also necessary, both to make the diagnosis and to follow treatment. An X-ray is usually taken to confirm the diagnosis and again to check the effectiveness of treatment. Most of the time you can expect to recover from a bout of pneumonia, even though it may take a little longer than antici-pated. There will usually be a gradual decrease in your temper-ature, but this is often less rapid than in younger persons. Cough and phlegm also may persist for a longer period. As dehydration is corrected and the fever subsides, the mental confusion that often accompanies the illness usually clears. You will gradually feel better and your appetite will return. You may feel weak and tired for weeks afterward, but this will pass. Ultimately, you should return to the state of health that you enjoyed prior to the illness.

Should all cases of pneumonia be treated?

In many ways the treatment of pneumonia presents a moral and ethical dilemma for the physician and families of older people. Some feel that nature should be allowed to take its course. With modern techniques and antibiotics, most older people will improve with treatment. The choice is usually not how to treat, but whether to treat, and this depends on the state of the individual's mental and physical health before the infection occurred.

If before the pneumonia developed you were functioning at a reasonable level, most physicians and families agree that treatment is appropriate. But sometimes the pneumonia is part of the final illness. For example, in the last stages of terminal cancer, pneumonia may indeed be "the friend of the aged." Before assuming this, a careful and full examination of your circumstances must be made. This will prevent effective therapy from being unnecessarily withheld or given to you when you should be allowed to die peacefully. But your wishes should be considered before decisions are made for you by your family or physician.

You should make it clear to your family and physician what type of treatment you would like should you become too ill to let your wishes be known. If you would prefer to let nature take its course, discuss this with them before you become ill.

TUBERCULOSIS

Tuberculosis, which is caused by a most unusual bacterium, was common in the nineteenth century and during the early decades of this century. Often, it resulted in death. Many great novels were written about artists, writers, and laborers who died from "consumption." Because of this reputation, tuberculosis always struck fear in everyone's heart. With improved sanitation and living conditions, however, the disease became less common.

Unlike other bacteria, the one causing tuberculosis grows slowly. Many older people were infected with it when they were young. If their health was otherwise good, most people had the strength to resist it, and they recovered. However, despite recovery, the bacteria lies dormant in the body, often in the lungs. During the later years, as the defense system deteriorates, they may become revitalized and begin to multiply and cause an active tuberculosis infection.

Sometimes the illness occurs in people who have poorly controlled diabetes mellitus. If another serious illness such as cancer exists, tuberculosis bacteria may cause an infection. The use of cortisone for diseases such as arthritis is sometimes responsible for allowing the bacteria to revitalize. Therefore, the illness usually occurs in an older person who was initially an immigrant or who lived in a city, and is suffering from a serious chronic illness or has been receiving cortisone.

What are the symptoms?

The most common place for tuberculosis to occur is in the lungs. You may experience cough, fever, and phlegm, just like in bronchitis or pneumonia. Unlike the other causes of chest infections, tuberculosis does not respond to the usual antibiotics. Your general health may deteriorate, and you may lose weight and your appetite and feel depressed. Occasionally, you may cough up blood. A persistent low-grade fever also is a common symptom.

A tuberculosis infection can also affect the kidneys, bowel, brain, liver, and bones. The diagnosis is often missed early in the illness because the physician often suspects other infections or malignancies first. One test that is often confusing is the *tuberculosis skin test*. When this is positive, it means that you have been exposed to tuberculosis bacteria at some time in your life. Many perfectly healthy people have a positive skin test, so it does not necessarily mean that you have an *active* infection. The degree of positivity varies. The more positive the test, the more likely is the presence of an infection.

How is the diagnosis made?

It may take many weeks before a diagnosis can be made. Your physician will analyze your sputum if you have a cough. In the absence of a cough, bronchial washings from a *bronchoscopy* or a biopsy of the bone marrow and liver may be necessary. A chest X-ray is helpful in making a diagnosis. Sometimes, despite many tests, including bacteriological cultures, X-rays, and scans, a definite diagnosis cannot be made. A trial course of antituberculosis drugs such as *isoniazid, ethambutol,* and *rifampin* may be started without a firm diagnosis. The results of this therapy may be all that there is to confirm the suspicion of tuberculosis. If you get better, it can be assumed that your infection was tuberculosis, because no other disease would respond to these special antituberculosis medications.

One elderly gentleman was brought to the hospital in a coma after having been treated for a few weeks with antibiotics for a bout of "bronchitis." His condition did not improve despite changing antibiotics, and his mental state was clouded by fever. Tests were done, and he was treated with potent antibiotics while the results of the tests were being awaited. Because of his coma, a *lumbar puncture* (spinal tap) was done, in which *cerebrospinal fluid* surrounding his brain and spinal cord was removed through a fine needle inserted into his back. Analysis of this fluid suggested tuberculosis affecting the brain. However, no actual bacteria were found on the bacteriological examination.

His poor response to potent antibiotics and a very positive tuberculosis skin test influenced the decision to start antituberculosis drugs. Within forty-eight hours his fever subsided and his level of consciousness improved. Four weeks later, he was sent home. He had survived a tuberculosis infection of his nervous system (tuberculosis meningitis). His dramatic response to antituberculosis therapy clinched the diagnosis.

Is tuberculosis curable?

Unlike many years ago, when "consumption" was a scourge, most cases of tuberculosis today, even in the very elderly, are curable. The treatment continues for twelve to eighteen months and in the majority of cases can be done at home with normal activities. Rarely is it necessary to enter a sanitorium for therapy. If treatment is stopped sooner, the disease can recur. Some people may have difficulties with a few of the newer drugs, and changes will have to be made. Your physician will supervise the medications and, with the help of blood tests, determine whether there are toxic side effects. Other members of your family should see a physician to make sure they have not contracted the illness.

URINARY TRACT INFECTIONS

The urinary tract includes the *kidneys*, the *bladder*, the *ureters*, which connect the kidneys to the bladder, and the *urethra*, which allows urine to be voided. In women the urethra is located just above the vagina. In men the urethra enters the penis after it passes through the prostate gland. The kidneys filter the blood and remove waste products from the body.

Most people empty their bladders four or five times daily, depending on their bladder capacity and the amount of fluid, including tea, coffee, and alcohol that they drink. Many kidney illnesses and drugs increase the need to urinate.

One common problem affecting the urinary tract in older people is infection. These infections should be treated immediately, not only because of the great discomfort they produce but also because of the serious illnesses they lead to.

Why are urinary tract infections so common?

Your normal defenses against infection decrease as you grow older. Also, kidney or bladder stones prevent all the urine from being emptied, and the urinary tract can become a source of repeated infections.

As men grow older, they often develop an enlargement of the prostate gland, which can interfere with the complete emptying of the bladder. Some urine remains in the bladder and be-

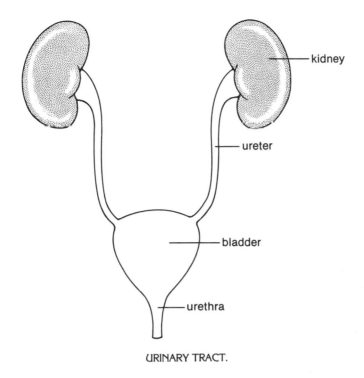

URINARY TRACT.

comes stagnant, and within weeks or months it becomes infected. Although antibiotics may help, the infection often returns, because the urine that normally helps to wash out bacteria collects in the bladder instead.

Some women develop a weakness in the muscles around their vagina, and the bladder begins to sag through the vaginal wall, creating a pouch *(cystocele)*. Urine becomes stagnant and an infection develops.

The *urethra* occasionally becomes narrowed and prevents complete bladder emptying. Treatment usually consists of widening the urethra with the assistance of instruments inserted under local anesthesia that gradually dilate it. This is often successful in decreasing the susceptibility to repeated urinary tract infections in some older women.

Some people with severe neurological diseases may lose control of their bladder. In such circumstances *catheters* (plastic tubes) may be inserted to keep urine from leaking and harming the skin. Tests can determine if the catheter is necessary before it is left in permanently. A permanent urinary catheter increases the risk of infection, although special precautions are taken to prevent this. However, sometimes its use is unavoidable. Even without the catheter, a person with a severe neurological disease is at risk of a urinary tract infection because of incomplete emptying of the bladder.

If you have diabetes mellitus or take large doses of painkillers (analgesics), there is a greater hazard of developing a urinary tract infection. With your doctor's advice, try to control your blood and urine sugar levels and avoid excessive amounts of analgesics.

What is the treatment for urinary tract infections?

Different types of bacteria cause infection of the urinary tract, but the degree of infection is also important. Some infections are potentially dangerous and require immediate, thorough treatment. Other types are chronic and may not consistently respond to antibiotic therapy or even need to be treated.

An acute infection can be dangerous. It may be complicated by a blood infection *(septicemia)*, which can cause severe illness. In these circumstances immediate treatment is important, usually consisting of intravenous fluids and potent antibiotics and other medications to help you through the danger period. In milder cases large amounts of fluids by mouth and antibiotics may be sufficient and treatment at home may be successful.

In some acute urinary tract infections, the illness is so severe that symptoms pointing to the urinary tract as the source of infection may not be obvious. Most people with active urinary tract infections feel a burning when they pass urine. It is often necessary to run to the bathroom urgently and frequently. But sometimes these symptoms are not experienced. Instead, one may become mentally confused, develop fever, and sometimes cease to pass urine altogether or in small amounts. This can result from the kidneys being severely infected or the bladder being blocked by an enlarged prostate.

Urine and blood tests are necessary for a proper diagnosis, and treatment is usually effective. Following therapy for a severe illness, your physician will determine if something can be done to prevent further attacks. He may recommend treatment for the prostate or repair of the cystocoele.

Some people may have bacteria growing in their urine but have no symptoms of infection. This is especially the case if you have a catheter, or if you have a neurological disease. There is a difference of opinion as to whether these infections need to be treated with antibiotic therapy or if they can be left alone. Some physicians recommend drugs that act as antiseptics to help clear the urine. Other physicians use small doses of antibiotics to keep the number of bacteria low, and thereby prevent severe infections. It is usually not possible to clear up these *asymptomatic* urinary tract infections completely with strong antibiotics. These drugs should be reserved for a severe infection that requires potent therapy.

OTHER INFECTIONS

SEPTICEMIA (BLOOD POISONING)

Bacteria can enter the bloodstream from many sources. As you grow older, your decreased defenses may allow bacteria to grow more easily in your body. The most common sources of septicemia are infections in other organs, including the liver, gallbladder, urinary tract, skin, and lungs. The symptoms are usually those of infection, with fever, mental confusion, and chills. If the infection comes from the urinary tract or lungs, you may have urinary burning or cough.

Is treatment effective?

Although septicemia is a potentially life-threatening illness, it can be treated in most cases. The outlook of the illness depends on its underlying cause and the state of your general health before the septicemia occurred. As well, some bacteria are easier to treat than others. You may go into shock and require hospitalization, intensive intravenous fluids, and antibiotic therapy. However, if you were well prior to the illness, there is a good chance for a complete recovery.

BACTERIAL ENDOCARDITIS

The lining of the heart, heart valves, and blood vessels is normally smooth, and bacteria that occasionally enter the bloodstream cannot find a place to settle. Also, the body's defenses usually clear them away. If you have suffered heart-valve damage because of rheumatic heart disease or just because of the aging process itself, the heart lining may no longer be smooth. Bacteria can settle on a valve, multiply, and then circulate in the blood to other parts of the body, causing subacute bacterial endocarditis (SBE).

The illness may follow a procedure such as dental work, surgery, or cystoscopy (looking into the bladder) in a person who has an abnormal valve or heart murmur. If the infection occurs a few weeks after the procedure, you may begin to feel weak and lose your appetite. You will probably develop a mild fever and sweating, especially at night. In severe cases bacteria may settle in the brain or kidneys and cause severe damage. In most instances this is rare during the early part of the illness.

A physician suspicious of this illness will take many blood tests, including *blood cultures*, to see if there are bacteria in your bloodstream. Since the bacteria are elusive, several blood samples are taken during the day and night in order to "catch" bacteria in at least one sample. This usually requires hospitalization.

Can bacterial endocarditis be prevented?

If you know that you have a diseased valve because you were told that you have a heart murmur, always inform your dentist and all physicians who look after you, because antibiotic treatment usually must precede and follow any dental treatment or surgery. Even vigorous cleaning of the teeth by a dental hygienist may require antibiotics before and after the procedure. In most cases bacterial endocarditis can be prevented with this antibiotic treatment. The risk is negligible. Penicillin is preferred, unless you are allergic to it.

Is the treatment for bacterial endocarditis always successful?

If the illness is diagnosed early, treatment is usually effective. However, on occasion there may already be damage to the brain, heart, or kidneys. The ultimate damage can be measured only after therapy is completed.

Intravenous antibiotics are used in large doses for a period of four to six weeks. During treatment blood tests will be done to measure whether the amount of antibiotic is sufficient to kill the bacteria and to clear the heart of infection. Although the treatment is long and tedious, it is usually successful.

If you have already suffered an attack of bacterial endocarditis, you are at a greater risk of a second episode. Therefore, you must make sure that you receive antibiotics whenever you have dental or surgical treatment. Preventive treatment must be started just *before* the dental work is begun and continued for two days after.

CELLULITIS (SKIN INFECTION)

Cellulitis, especially of a leg, is a common problem in the older person. It may follow an abrasion or other wound to the leg, face, or nose. If you have varicose veins, you may suffer from swelling of your legs. This extra fluid reduces the body's defense against infection. If bacteria enter your skin, they can become a source of infection and spread throughout a limb. In some cases cellulitis is complicated by blood poisoning (septicemia), which requires antibiotic therapy in large doses. Milder cases can be treated at home with antibiotics by mouth, local, gentle heat, and elevation of the affected leg.

ANTIBIOTIC TREATMENT

Antibiotics are produced by microorganisms, such as bacteria or fungi, that prevent the growth and multiplication of deleterious bacteria. Years ago it was discovered that this antibiotic material could be collected and purified and then used to kill harmful bacteria in humans.

Antibiotics today are manufactured in a number of ways. We can grow the special microorganisms and collect the antibiotic substance they produce. After purification the antibiotic can be used to treat illness. Many newer, important antibiotics are produced synthetically, a more efficient and cheaper method.

Drugs other than antibiotics also interfere with the growth and multiplication of harmful bacteria. They are called chemotherapeutic agents, and *sulfonamide* (usually called *sulfa*) is an important member of this group. It was developed before penicillin, the first antibiotic, and is still useful in certain types of infections. In general, most people use the word *antibiotic* to include all of these drugs.

There are many varieties of antibiotics, but no antibiotic is effective against every type of bacteria. In fact, this is good because the human body contains many useful, friendly bacteria and it could be dangerous if these were killed.

When should antibiotics be used?

Antibiotics are effective only in the treatment of infections caused by bacteria and some other more unusual germs. They are not at all effective in the treatment of illnesses caused by viruses, and they should not be used to treat the ordinary cold or flu, both of which are caused by viruses.

Some people think that an antibiotic can prevent a cold or flu from developing into a more serious bacterial infection. In fact, the antibiotic may damage normal bacteria and result in a disease more dangerous than the one for which it was unnecessarily taken.

Antibiotics should not be taken without the advice of a physician, and they should be used *only* after it has been clearly established that the illness is caused by bacteria. And they should not be reused at a later date without consulting a physician. Some antibiotics lose their effect with age or even become dangerous. Except under special circumstances, such as if you suffer from chronic bronchitis, and have prearranged a treatment program with your physician, self-medication with these drugs is potentially harmful. Often, a specimen of your throat, urine, or sputum will be examined before an antibiotic is prescribed.

One elderly lady began to experience fever and weakness a few weeks after she had dental surgery. Although she knew she had a heart murmur, she failed to mention this to the dental surgeon and therefore did not receive antibiotic therapy. When she eventually went to her own physician with a fever, she did not mention that she had received dental treatment a few weeks before. Her physician prescribed antibiotics because she had evidence of an infection in her urine. Within a few days she felt better and her fever improved. She stopped the antibiotics on her own.

About two weeks later she developed fever again and assumed that it was from the same infection. She took her remaining antibiotics without consulting her physician. Her fever decreased, and once again she felt well. A week later the fever returned. Fortunately, she had used all the antibiotics before and had to return to a physician, who found that she was suffering from bacterial endocarditis. The diagnosis and treatment had been unnecessarily delayed because she diagnosed and treated herself with antibiotics without medical supervision.

Can antibiotics have side effects?

As with all medications, antibiotics have potential side effects. It is very important for you to tell your physician about any problems you had with antibiotics in the past. Some people are allergic to certain types, and allergies to them can cause skin rashes and swelling of the face, among other symptoms. It is important to keep a record of these allergies. The physician can then choose a different antibiotic or at least take precautions to prevent problems if the antibiotic to which you are allergic has to be used.

A *Medic-Alert bracelet* should be worn if your allergy is dangerous. Some people, for example, are allergic to penicillin and develop severe breathing problems or go into shock. If by chance you are in an accident or lose consciousness, the bracelet will warn any physician of this allergy. It is also useful for all other allergies, serious illnesses or necessary drug treatments.

Some simple bracelets can be bought in most drugstores. There is also an international organization that issues special bracelets and keeps a record of your particular medical problem. Each of these *Medic-Alert* bracelets is numbered and coded. In an emergency, a physician can call the organization to find out about the medical problems that are listed on the bracelet. This can sometimes save your life.

Frequently, allergies to antibiotics are confused with other types of less dangerous side effects, such as nausea, drowsiness, or diarrhea. However, it is very important to understand the difference between an allergy and a side effect. Some people claim that they are allergic to every type of antibiotic, when in fact they have had only minor side effects. It can be very difficult for a physician to choose a proper antibiotic if you tell him that you are allergic to all antibiotics because you once became nauseated when you took one. Physicians are usually aware of the side effects, and they take precautions to prevent them. Usually, the need for therapy outweighs the relative risk of adverse side effects.

Why are antibiotics sometimes given by mouth and sometimes given by injection or intravenously?

The way antibiotics are given usually depends on the severity of the infection and your ability to take the drug by mouth. For mild infections the antibiotic is usually quite effective when taken as pills or syrup.

If the infection is serious or if you are in shock or are weak, treatment will be started with injections or intravenous therapy. It may be continued later by mouth. If extremely large doses of antibiotics are necessary, as in the case of blood poisoning or bacterial endocarditis, they are given intravenously.

CHAPTER 13

Genitourinary and Gynecological Disorders

The genitourinary system consists of the *kidneys, ureters, bladder,* and *urethra,* as well as the *organs of reproduction.* From the kidneys to the bladder, the urinary systems are exactly the same in men and women. In women the urethra has only a short distance to travel before it reaches the surface, just above the entrance to the vagina. Women's organs of reproduction are in close proximity within the pelvis to the bladder and urethra. Because of this, abnormalities of the urinary system can affect the organs of reproduction and vice versa.

In men the urethra must pass through the *prostate gland* and the *penis* before it exits from the body. Because the distance along which the urethra must pass is longer, the possibility of disorders is greater.

For most problems occurring in the male genitourinary system a *urologist* is consulted, whereas women would consult a *gynecologist.*

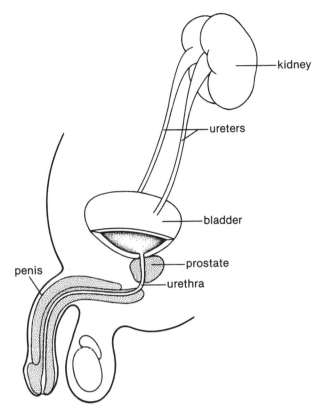

MALE GENITOURINARY TRACT.

KIDNEY DISEASE

Kidney problems occur in men and women. The two kidneys lie deep within the body on either side of the spine just below the diaphragm, the muscle that separates the abdomen and chest. Blood passes through the kidneys from the *renal (kidney) arteries*, and the kidneys filter the blood and remove waste products, which are dissolved in the urine. The kidneys have a great deal of reserve, and many people can live with one functioning kidney. Disorders can affect either one or both kidneys. When both are seriously damaged, waste products build up in the body.

The symptoms of kidney disease depend on the underlying cause. Some problems cause pain, which is usually felt in the loins (the small of the back) or in the side of the abdomen. This is common with kidney stones, which are often passed down the ureters. Stones may cause a pain that shoots into the groin as well as the back. Many kidney diseases are gradual in their development, and the symptoms are the result only of the accumulation of waste products in the blood. This process, called *kidney failure*, causes weakness, fatigue, and often anemia. Some people experience a metallic taste in the mouth, itching skin, and an increase or decrease in the amount of urine that is passed. When there is an increase, the urine is usually very pale in color and contains few waste products. If the condition continues without treatment, it can seriously affect your general health, especially your heart, blood pressure, and lungs.

Is kidney disease common in the elderly?

There are many reasons why some older people develop kidney problems. Repeated kidney infections over the years and inflammation *(nephritis)* can damage the kidneys. Sometimes these illnesses first develop in later years, or they started years before and gradually progress.

If you have a long history of high blood pressure, especially if it has not been controlled, or atherosclerosis, there can also be a gradual deterioration in kidney function. Small pieces of *atheroma* (fatty material) can become dislodged from renal (kidney) blood vessels and block the flow of blood to the kidneys, thereby causing injury. If you suffer from kidney stones that have not been successfully treated either by medication or surgical removal, they may partially block the ureters and kidneys and prevent the flow of urine, thus becoming a source of repeated infections. Unrelieved obstruction from an enlarged prostate can do the same.

The overuse of certain medications, such as analgesics (painkillers), can injure your kidneys, and this is true of some of the newer and stronger antibiotics as well. If you already have kidney damage, some antibiotics have to be used cautiously.

Tumors of the kidney, both benign and malignant, can occur in older people. They may show themselves either by growing and spreading to other parts of the body or by causing hemorrhage within the kidney. If you see blood in your urine, contact your physician immediately, even if the bleeding stops by itself.

Individuals with diabetes mellitus can develop kidney disease and are more prone to infection of the urinary tract. If you suffer from this disorder, your blood and urine should be examined at least every six months to check the function of your kidneys.

What special precautions should be taken if you have kidney disease?

You probably can manage quite well and be reasonably healthy even if your kidneys are not working completely normally. The types of kidney disease affecting older individuals may develop slowly and may not seriously affect your health unless progressive damage occurs. If you become severely ill or dehydrated, your kidneys may fail to work properly. Fluids often have to be taken intravenously to correct this problem.

Some drugs that are given for other illnesses can have deleterious effects on your kidneys. Your physician should alter the dosage of these drugs so as to decrease the chance of damaging your kidneys. Other drugs that the body normally gets rid of through the kidneys may accumulate to unsafe levels if you have kidney disease. Your physician will make frequent blood tests to ensure that they are not accumulating. Of special importance is the drug *digoxin*, which many older people need for heart disease. This medication can accumulate quickly in your blood. The earliest symptom is usually loss of appetite.

Sometimes the amount of digoxin in the blood must be measured before the proper dose can be determined.

PROSTATE PROBLEMS

The *prostate* is a plump doughnut-shaped gland surrounding the lower part of the *urethra* just before it enters the penis. It produces the *prostatic fluid* that helps carry and nourish sperm during ejaculation. As men grow older, the prostate often increases in size and compresses the urethra, causing the diameter of the passage to get smaller and thus preventing the normal passage of urine. Because the bladder cannot empty completely, the urine collects and causes back pressure on the kidneys. The ability of the kidneys to work properly will be reduced, and if left untreated, the condition can lead to kidney damage.

You may not be immediately aware of the urine buildup but might notice some difficulty in passing urine, or it may take longer to start urinating and the stream may lose its force. You may dribble urine or find that you have to get up at night to urinate. Some people lose control completely. In some cases the urine flow may stop completely. You will probably seek immediate attention because of pain in your lower abdomen. In other cases progress is so gradual that you may not become aware of the problem until you develop other symptoms. A rectal exam may reveal an enlarged prostate. However, before a definite diagnosis is made, it is usually necessary to do a *cystoscopic* examination, in which a tube, passed into the bladder through the penis, examines the prostate and bladder.

Can prostate disease be malignant?

In most instances enlargement of the prostate gland is the result of a benign process. The disease does not spread to other parts of the body, and once treated it usually does not recur. Sometimes a second treatment many years later is required.

How is prostate enlargement treated?

When there are symptoms of incomplete bladder emptying, the blockage must be relieved. This is usually done by surgery through the abdomen or through the penis *(transurethral resection,* or *TURP)*. Even very elderly men can usually withstand prostate surgery that is done through the penis. You should not refuse this operation because of your age. It is not a difficult procedure, and it is usually successful in relieving symptoms. In very frail individuals, it can be done with a spinal anesthetic.

Rarely are there problems after a transurethral resection. You may temporarily lose some control of your urine, but this is usually not permanent unless a neurological problem was present before surgery. There is usually no interference with sexual abilities. In fact, your sexual capabilities may improve, because the excess pressure in the bladder and kidneys may have interfered with normal sexual function.

What kinds of tumors can affect the prostate?

Some people develop a malignant tumor (cancer of the prostate). This is often found accidentally during surgery for benign prostate obstruction. In most instances the tumor is usually small and limited to the prostate itself. In many such cases it will not spread elsewhere. However, there may be evidence that the cancer spread to the bladder, liver, and bones before the diagnosis of the original tumor is made.

Can cancer of the prostate be cured?

If your prostate gland is removed while the tumor is small, the malignancy may not have spread. If the tumor has already expanded, surgical removal of the testicles, which eliminates the male hormones that the tumor needs to grow, can halt its progress. Various medications, including female hormones, are often also helpful. Radiation to the prostate or to painful areas of invaded bone are sometimes useful. The malignancy may take years to progress if it is treated energetically. You can often enjoy years of comfort and health with proper medical management.

BLADDER DISORDERS

The bladder can store sufficient quantities of urine so that you normally have to empty it only four or five times a day. It receives its stimulus to empty by nerves that come from the spinal cord and which are partially controlled by the brain.

The bladder can be injured by urinary tract diseases, or by illnesses that interfere with its ability to empty completely and efficiently. When your bladder is not working properly, your health as well as your social life can be severely affected. Men and women have slightly different bladder disorders, but the results are often similar.

What bladder problems do men develop?

If you suffer from prostate enlargement, you may develop an overstretched bladder until the blockage is corrected. If this is done early enough, your bladder can be retrained and made to work efficiently and normally again.

Some people of both sexes develop bladder tumors. These usually become evident when blood is seen in the urine. The color of the urine may be bright red or lightly wine colored. Although some of these tumors may be malignant and can spread, many of them are benign or minimally malignant. They can often be treated by passing a cystoscope into the bladder through the urethra and *burning (fulgurating)* them. The earlier the tumors are treated, the better the result. Whenever you see blood in your urine, report it to your physician immediately.

Only occasionally are the tumors malignant. In this case the bladder may have to be removed and a "new bladder" made out of a piece of intestine. Such a procedure is usually done by a urologist, and it is often successful, especially if the tumor has not spread from the bladder to other parts of the body. Radiation can also be used successfully.

Why does the bladder "fall down" in some older women?

Women who have had many pregnancies may develop a weakness of the pelvic muscles that surround the vagina. Being overweight aggravates the problem. In such cases the bladder protrudes into the vagina and causes a feeling that something is "falling down," dragging, or pressing, especially when you are standing or walking. This is called a *cystocoele* or *prolapse.*

The cystocoele may cause you to suffer from *"stress" incontinence*, which means that you lose control of your urine when you laugh, cough, sneeze, or strain yourself, as when pushing or carrying heavy items. You will be more likely to develop infections of your bladder urine if the cystocoele is fairly large and the urine stagnates because it is not completely emptied.

The condition is treated by a gynecologist, either through the use of a *pessary*, a synthetic device that holds the bladder in place, or a surgical repair.

What is a urethral stricture?

In men the urethra passes through the penis, and in women it exits just above the vagina. The urethra can become narrowed in both men and women and the results are similar. This sometimes occurs after injury, childbirth, prostate surgery, or following infection. Urine builds up in the bladder and stretches it. This increases the tendency to infection and may lead to difficulties in passing urine or incontinence.

Diagnosis usually depends on a cystoscopy. Treatment consists of dilating the urethra gradually by passing instruments of increasingly large diameters through it. Sometimes treatment must be repeated periodically. Symptoms are often successfully controlled with this therapy.

URINARY INCONTINENCE

Urinary incontinence, or loss of urine control, can have a terrible effect on self-esteem and the ability to remain at home and socialize normally. Families often have great difficulty in dealing with an incontinent spouse or parent, and institutionalization may be decided upon if the incontinence cannot be tolerated or managed.

Is urinary incontinence
a natural consequence of aging?

Urinary incontinence is not a result of aging, but of disease. One common cause in men is prostate enlargement, where the loss of urine is the result of an overflow from an excessively distended bladder. Surgery to remove the obstruction is usually successful. Some men develop a narrowing of their urethra, sometimes as a result of past prostate surgery. It can usually be corrected by surgery or by gradually widening the urethra. Women may develop incontinence because of a cystocoele or an inflammation of the urethra known as a *caruncle*.

Both men and women can suffer from bladder infections, which may lead to urgency, frequent urination, and incontinence. You may or may not experience burning urination, especially if the infection has existed for a long time.

Many drugs can lead to urinary incontinence. The fast-acting diuretics that are given for high blood pressure or heart failure can quickly produce so much urine that you may not reach the bathroom in time. This may look like urinary incontinence but is not really a bladder problem. Many sedatives and tranquilizers can make you groggy and lead to incontinence because you are too drowsy to go to the bathroom or do not feel the urge to.

Those who have suffered brain damage from strokes or dementia may experience urinary incontinence. This is a common cause of this problem and one of the most difficult to treat. Diseases that affect the nerves controlling the bladder may also lead to urinary incontinence. Nerves can be damaged by diabetes mellitus or an unrecognized case of syphilis from many years before. Back injuries or diseases that affect the spinal cord can also produce this condition.

What tests can be done to diagnose the cause of urinary incontinence?

Measurements of your kidney function and tests to reveal urine infection are usually done. A kidney X-ray (*intravenous pyelogram*) may be necessary to show if there is kidney damage or a blockage of the bladder.

If the cause of incontinence is not immediately clear, a *cystometrogram* is often used to measure the amount of urine that your bladder can hold and whether the nerves controlling it are functioning well. During the test, increasing quantities of sterile fluids are put into your bladder and the pressure developed within it is measured. The test determines whether your bladder is contracting (emptying) normally.

Are catheters a good treatment for urinary incontinence?

A urinary catheter (plastic tube) allows urine to drain from the bladder into a plastic bag, and it may be useful in temporarily relieving a blocked bladder. It is not the best treatment for urinary incontinence because it can cause infection. Catheters should be reserved for those who cannot otherwise be treated and in whom the risk of urinary infection is outweighed by the need to be kept completely dry. For instance, after major surgery or trauma, or if there are pressure sores, urinary incontinence may contaminate wounds or macerate the skin.

What other treatments are available?

If a urinary infection is found, it may be playing a role in urinary incontinence. The infection should be treated with antibiotics or with drugs that decrease the frequency and urge to urinate. Some people become incontinent as part of a depressive illness, and treatment with antidepressant medications can show a remarkable improvement. The use of diuretics and sedatives should be evaluated and, whenever possible, decreased or discontinued.

Incontinence in men can be controlled by a clamp that closes the penis. This is rather uncomfortable, and one must be mentally alert for it to be applied properly. In most instances it should be avoided. A condomlike sheath that covers the penis and is connected to a bag by plastic tubing is sometimes useful, especially at night. However, this often causes irritation of the penis.

For those people who are partially or completely bedridden, incontinence pads have been specially designed to absorb urine but leave the body relatively dry. For those who are more mobile, there are special undergarments that absorb urine but prevent the skin from becoming wet. Disposable diapers for infants or toddlers work the same way and can be put inside underpants. They can be very useful in the occasionally incontinent person who is mobile at home or in an institution.

Some improvement can follow changes in habits. Women's symptoms may improve if they lean forward when passing urine. This helps empty the bladder more efficiently. Although the standing position is normal for men, some can pass urine more easily sitting down.

You should try to pass your urine frequently. A commode by the bed or a urinal used every few hours may help avoid bed or undergarment wetting. Whenever possible, you should remain mobile and stay out of bed. If you have severe constipation, you may develop urinary incontinence until your bowel is cleared. The rectum should be examined to be sure that a full bowel is not pressing on your bladder.

Sometimes incontinence results from a neurological disease, particularly brain tumors and in an unusual type of *hydro-cephalus,* occasionally found in the elderly. A neurologist can make these diagnoses. Surgical treatment of the brain disorder in these unusual situations may also improve the incontinence.

GYNECOLOGICAL PROBLEMS

The gynecological organs include the *ovaries*, where during fertile years ova (eggs) are produced, the *fallopian tubes*, and the *uterus* (womb). At the lower end of the uterus is the *cervix*, which protrudes into the *vagina*. The cervix has an opening to allow menstrual blood (or babies) to pass from the uterus. The vagina contains a special lining that is kept smooth and supple by female hormones. Its many glands produce a lubricating fluid during sexual excitement. The *clitoris*, which elicits sexual pleasure when stimulated, lies just above the entrance to the vagina. The *vulva* is the fold of skin that encloses the vagina.

Most women have a menstrual cycle that starts sometime in their early teens. During fertile years periods are more or less regular but gradually become irregular as *menopause* approaches; or they may have been regular until menopause, when they suddenly stop. At the time of menopause, you may have experienced a combination of uncomfortable symptoms, including hot flashes with sweating, headaches, depression, and sleep disturbances. You may have been given female replacement hormones, which probably modified the symptoms and

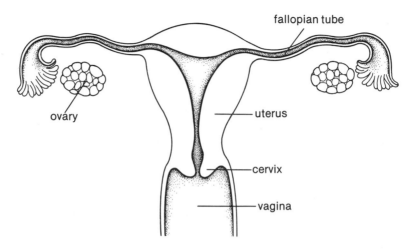

FEMALE REPRODUCTIVE SYSTEM.

returned you to a feeling of well-being. Some women have no discomfort at all during menopause.

You may feel that once you have stopped being sexually active, you should no longer have any problems with your gynecological system. You, and perhaps your physician, may adopt a "no use—no look" approach. But as you grow older, you are just as likely to develop gynecological problems, and they should not be neglected. A pelvic examination and a *"Pap" smear* should be part of your routine annual checkup.

FEMALE REPLACEMENT HORMONES

If the symptoms that you experienced during menopause were severe, it is possible that you were given female replacement hormones *(estrogen)*. It may be years since you started taking these pills which probably improved your physical and mental health enormously. There have been some suggestions lately, however, which are far from resolved, that prolonged use of these hormones may increase the chance of uterine cancer. Some physicians feel that by adding a second female hormone

294

(progesterone) to the original hormone, the risk decreases and perhaps there is even a positive benefit.

There may be a number of other positive aspects to the long-term use of female hormones during postmenopausal years. There is some suggestion that your bones may not weaken as quickly, your skin may hold its elasticity and have better tone, and your vagina will not be as prone to infection, dryness, and itching. Some women cannot tolerate the hormones because of bloating, weight gain, nausea, and vaginal bleeding.

Because hormone treatment is controversial, some physicians recommend that women should try to reduce the amount they take and then discontinue it altogether. If you can do this without great discomfort, it is probably worthwhile until the risks are proven or disproven. If, however, you cannot, you should take the smallest amount of medication that makes you comfortable and consult your physician or a gynecologist about adding small quantities of a second progesterone hormone to the estrogen. The drugs should also be taken in cycles, with "rest" periods between medication, rather than on a continuous basis (usually three weeks "on" and one week "off"). A gynecological exam every six to twelve months is important if you take these hormone medications.

VAGINAL BLEEDING

Many women are afraid to admit that they have vaginal bleeding so long after their periods have stopped. If the bleeding stops by itself, you may postpone consulting your physician. If you use female hormones, bleeding may occasionally occur as a result. However, there may be other, more serious causes of bleeding even if you take these hormones. In all cases you should report any bleeding or any change in amount of bleeding or predictability to your doctor.

Sometimes the wall of the vagina becomes thin because of a lack of hormonal (estrogen) stimulation and causes bleeding, itching, or irritation. This is called *senile vaginitis.* Often a small amount of estrogen cream applied to the area will relieve the symptoms.

An important cause of bleeding is the presence of tumors, either benign or malignant. Unless the cause is obvious from a gynecological examination, many physicians will recommend a *dilatation and curettage (D & C)* to diagnose the cause and ensure that no tumors are present. The *D & C* consists of widening the entrance of the cervix while you are anesthetized and "scraping" the lining of the uterus to obtain tissue for analysis. With this procedure the cause of the bleeding can usually be identified and proper treatment recommended.

VAGINAL ITCHING AND PAIN

Vaginal itching can be very embarrassing, and you may even be afraid to leave your home in order to avoid scratching yourself in public. You may be ashamed to approach your physician for the same reasons that you may not admit to vaginal bleeding.

A number of infections cause vaginal itching. A common one is the result of a yeast called *Candida albicans.* This may be the first sign of diabetes mellitus. Infections of the urinary tract may also cause local irritation, but this is more common if you have some urinary incontinence. *Senile vaginitis* may cause itching and pain in addition to bleeding, but it usually responds to local treatment with estrogen cream. Other skin problems in the vaginal area can be easily diagnosed and treated.

PROLAPSE

A prolapse is a weakening of the vaginal wall that causes the bladder to sag into the vagina. The most common symptoms are a fullness or heaviness in the vaginal area and a leakage of urine when coughing or straining. There may be an increased susceptibility to urinary tract infections. Sometimes part of the intestine may protrude into the vagina and also cause problems with bowel movements.

In many instances surgical repair of a prolapse is the most effective treatment to relieve your symptoms completely. If you are fearful of surgery or have other medical problems, a *pessary* may be successful. This is a doughnut-shaped synthetic device that Is put Into the vagina to keep the prolapse from sagging.

TUMORS

Age does not protect you from developing a malignant gynecological growth. Malignant tumors of the cervix, uterus, and ovaries can occur at any age. The symptoms may be that of vaginal bleeding or vague symptoms such as weight loss and abdominal swelling.

Treatment is usually directed by a gynecologist and on-cologist (cancer specialist). This may include surgery, radiation, and chemotherapy, or a combination of any of these treat-ments. Many women respond very well to such treatment. If your physician feels that this therapy may succeed, it should not be refused because of your age.

VAGINAL ODOR

Some women are aware of an offensive odor in their vaginal area. This can be associated with a vaginal discharge, but the most common causes are various infections, such as that of the yeast *Candida albicans*, often associated with diabetes mellitus. Perspiration from poor hygiene and excess fat may exaggerate the odor.

Occasionally a tumor in the vulva, vagina, cervix, or uterus produces a foul-smelling discharge which may contain blood. Such a discharge is not normal, and you should consult your physician about it immediately.

CHAPTER 14

Neoplastic Disease: Tumors, Growths, and Cancer

Sometimes cells in the body grow and multiply without listening to the body's commands. The result is a *tumor*, either *benign* or *malignant*. Benign tumors do not spread to other parts of the body, but they cause damage by pushing aside and pressing on neighboring tissues and organs. Malignant tumors invade adjacent tissues and also break off and spread to different parts of the body. These distant malignant cells are called *metastates*, and the process is *metastatic spread*.

Cancer, or *carcinoma*, is not a single disease but an all-inclusive term to describe the many varieties of malignant tumors. The word is often used too loosely and usually strikes fear into the hearts of most people, young and old. I have heard patients with severe life-threatening heart disease ask if they had cancer. When they were told that they did not, they said, "Thank God, it's not cancer," even though their heart disease was in many ways more dangerous.

Certain types of malignancies are found more often in older people, and others are found more commonly in the young.

Since time is one factor that allows malignant tumors to grow, it is understandable that if you are older you will have a greater chance of developing a malignant growth than a younger person. This does not mean that age causes cancer, and it does not imply that it is inevitable. Depending on the organ involved, the treatment and response will vary. The types of treatment for cancer change rapidly, so some more malignant tumors might improve temporarily with newer forms of therapy. An *oncologist* (cancer specialist) should be consulted for advice as to the likelihood of the various treatments being effective.

What kind of treatments are available for cancer?

Surgery serves a number of important purposes. A malignant growth may be removed completely, before it has damaged neighboring tissues or has spread to other parts of the body. When this is successful, the cancer may be cured and never return again. It may even be beneficial to operate on a tumor that has spread to other parts of the body. If the tumor causes symptoms because of pressure on neighboring organs, or if it causes a blockage of the intestinal or urinary tract, its removal may greatly relieve uncomfortable symptoms. Other treatments are more effective when the size of the tumor is reduced through surgery.

Another important type of treatment is *radiation therapy*, in which beams of high-energy radiation are focused on tumors or collections of malignant cells. This is often effective in killing the malignant growth or decreasing its speed of development. Radiation can harm healthy tissue, so lead shields and special focusing devices are used, usually successfully, to prevent it from being damaged.

Radiation therapy is sometimes used in conjunction with surgery and drug therapy. After the tumor is removed, radiation can decrease the likelihood of malignant cells spreading from the original site of the growth.

Treatment with various medications, called *chemotherapeutic agents*, can interfere with the growth and development of many kinds of tumors. They are used with radiation therapy, with surgery, or often alone. *Combination chemotherapy*, or a combination of drugs, can be beneficial because different varieties of medications can attack the tumor in different places. Also, a smaller amount of each may be effective, thereby decreasing their side effects. And the malignancy may regress more quickly if different parts of its growth are attacked separately.

In addition to chemotherapy, some cancers will improve with *hormone therapy.* Some tumors need either male or female hormones to grow. Changes in the amount of these hormones in the body may decrease the speed with which the tumors develop. Hormones are sometimes used with surgery, with radiation therapy, and occasionally with other drugs.

One of the major problems with radiation and drug therapy are side effects or complications. Even with the best methods available, it is difficult to kill malignant cells without harming normal cells. Whenever possible, physicians try to decrease the possibility or duration of side effects without compromising the benefits of therapy. Some side effects are uncomfortable but not dangerous; others are so severe that they interfere with further treatments.

When cancer treatment is begun, you and your physician should discuss fully the likely side effects. Even though they may be uncomfortable, it is more likely that you will accept them if you know about them beforehand, rather than finding out after the treatment has begun. For instance, if you know that you may temporarily lose your hair following chemotherapy or radiation therapy, you might buy a wig before treatment is begun. This will allow you and others to get used to the way you look in a wig.

Many side effects are transient and can be prevented by taking certain medications before the therapy is begun. A period of trial and error may be necessary before your physician can prevent some of the common, minor side effects, such as nausea or vomiting, whenever you receive chemotherapy. Usually, the side effects can be controlled.

Is treatment effective?

It is often assumed by families and members of the medical profession that once a diagnosis of cancer is made, the older person should be allowed to "die in peace." This is unfair, because many individuals will respond well to anticancer treatment. No one should have to develop a bowel blockage because of cancer in order to avoid surgery. Usually surgery to relieve a blockage can be performed without great danger.

Although in most instances the cancer will not be cured, you may feel a significant improvement in your symptoms and have your life prolonged in a comfortable manner. No one should be deprived of these benefits because of age. It is interesting that malignancy in older people often progresses very slowly. Who is to say that, during the extra time therapy gives you, some major event may not occur in your life or a new form of treatment may not be found for your disease?

Will cancer return after treatment?

Although many malignancies will respond to treatment for a period of time, quite often the disease returns. This does not mean that a second course of treatment will not be successful, especially since new types of treatment are constantly being discovered.

Should you be told that you have cancer?

This is one of the most difficult questions that physicians and families face. I believe that it is usually beneficial for you to know what is happening to your life. Most people are far stronger than their families and physicians believe. You should have the right to know about your problem so that you can make appropriate plans for your future.

However, you should be told with tact and care. Often a physician can assess just how much you really want to know about your illness. He may gradually unfold the "full truth" to you as confidence between the two of you grows.

An elderly lady that I looked after had metastatic lung cancer. She had fluid in the lung spaces *(pleural effusion)* and had difficulty breathing. Her children begged me not to tell her of her disease because "it would kill her" if she knew. With reluctance, I agreed to call the illness a type of "inflammation."

A number of treatments to prevent the lung fluid from reaccumulating were tried. Unfortunately, they were not successful. The woman became more and more ill and every day asked me, "What kind of illness is this that makes the fluid return?" I answered, "It is a type of inflammation." One day, when she was gravely ill, she said to me, "This illness is worse than cancer, because with cancer at least you know what you're dealing with. This one is a real mystery." She died not long after this.

Because of their inability to discuss the problem with their mother, her children were not able to face the likelihood of her death. And she was not able to make the kind of honest decisions that people may want to make when they know they do not have much more time in this world. Thus it is essential that you discuss with your family and your physician how much you would like to know should you become ill. And it is best to discuss this while you are healthy, rather than waiting until a serious illness occurs.

Any organ of the body can be affected by malignant disease. Some varieties of cancer are more common than others, and as you grow older, certain classes of tumors may occur more frequently. Depending on the part of the body involved, the signs of the disease can differ and the kinds of treatment and their likelihood of success vary.

LUNG CANCER

A great deal has been written about lung cancer. Almost everyone knows that a strong association exists between lung cancer and cigarette smoking. However, one often hears the rationalization, "Mr. X died of lung cancer and he never smoked in his life."

There are, in fact, a number of varieties of lung cancer. Those that originate in the lung have a very high correlation with cigarette smoking. Although an unusual type of lung tumor is sometimes found in older individuals who have never smoked, in general those who have smoked heavily for many years are the most susceptible.

Cancer from another part of the body can eventually *spread* to the lungs as *metastases.* This of course has nothing to do with smoking and may be one of the reasons that people have the impression that nonsmokers run the same risk of getting lung cancer as smokers. This is not so. If you smoke, your chances of getting lung cancer are many times higher than if you do not. It is too late to stop after you already have the disease. How often I have heard the lament, "I'll never touch another cigarette," when it was no longer of any use.

Of the varieties of lung cancer associated with smoking, some are more lethal than others. If the diagnosis is made after symptoms of cancer have begun, the possibility of cure is small. An increase in the amount of cough or recurring chest infections are warning signs that something more serious than a simple infection is involved. The expectoration of blood may be the first sign of lung cancer. Weight loss, impairment of appetite, or undue fatigue may be early symptoms. Sometimes the illness first presents itself because it has already spread to other parts of the body, such as the brain or bones. Headaches, weakness of limbs, or fractures for no apparent reason may be manifestations of the disease.

If the illness is discovered early (as may be the case if it is found accidentally during a routine chest X-ray), treatment has a better chance of being successful. The first suspicion of the disease may be an X-ray that reveals a "shadow," in which case the physician will take a sputum sample to see if the cells are abnormal. It may be necessary to perform a *bronchoscopy* and *biopsy* to see if a tumor is present and if it has spread. Very often, if surgery is considered, many X-rays and scans will be done to ensure that the cancer has not spread to other parts of the body.

The results may show no evidence of tumor spread, and the growth may be small. Especially if found by chance, there is a possibility that in some types of lung tumors surgical removal of part of the lung may be successful in curing the disease. Unfortunately, many people with lung cancer also have chronic bronchitis and emphysema, which makes surgery more hazardous.

In some instances surgery can be successfully performed, and occasionally it completely removes the tumor. All factors must be taken into account first, including the kind of cancer, the evidence of spread to other parts of the body, and the general health of the patient. But surgery should not be discarded as a possibility because of age alone.

BREAST CANCER

Breast cancer is the most common malignancy in women. Although its exact cause is not clear, it appears to be partially hereditary. Whether hormones such as birth control pills or those taken after menopause play any role in causing breast cancer has not yet been proven.

Breast cancer is often noticed by chance, either by the woman herself or by her husband or physician. Self-examination, a method that all women should learn, can reveal small lumps, which may be the first sign of breast cancer. If you notice a lump in your breast, consult your physician immediately. Never assume that if you ignore it, it will go away by itself. If you are not certain how to examine your breasts by yourself, you can ask your physician for instruction. Many breast clinics are available for examinations and advice of this type. There are also brochures distributed by national cancer societies that explain breast self-examination.

Benign tumors of the breast are more common in younger women. The chances are therefore greater that, with increasing age, if you find a lump, it will require surgical removal. Many physicians will do special X-rays of the breast *(mammograms)* to determine if the lump has the appearance of a malignant tumor. Sometimes a needle is put into the lump under local anesthetic and some cells removed. This may reveal that the lump is in fact a cyst (collection of fluid) and not a tumor. In all cases, if a lump is found, it should be fully investigated and surgery considered if it is likely to be malignant.

Because breast cancer metastasizes (spreads), the tumor should be removed as soon as possible. The physician will also make sure that, if malignant, it has not spread. This is done before surgery by the use of X-rays and scans and during surgery by examining the tissues surrounding the tumor.

There appears to be little evidence that a radical mastectomy, in which underlying muscles and lymph nodes are removed along with the diseased breast, gives any real benefit to women with breast cancer. Especially in older women, the operation that seems most appropriate is the removal of the breast alone and the *lymph nodes* that drain the breast. In certain cases the removal of the cancerous lump, without the whole breast, may be sufficient, particularly in the very elderly, who may not as readily withstand a longer, more strenuous operation. This is often called a *lumpectomy*.

Some patients receive radiation treatment in addition to surgery, whereas others are treated with radiation alone. Sometimes radiation therapy is not given at the time of surgery but is used only if there is evidence that the tumor has recurred. The results of the different treatments are controversial, and it is still not clear what method is best for all women. If the tumor has spread to other parts of the body, there may be a good response to various hormones. Radiation treatment to bones that may be painful because of invasion by the tumor can be helpful in relieving symptoms. In some instances chemotherapy is of value.

Although breast cancer is a serious disease, in older women its progress and spread can be very slow. Many older women have survived surgery and have done very well for many years without any evidence of a recurrence. Others, although the cancer spread, respond extremely well to the newer hormonal treatments and live comfortably for many years. With proper treatment, the chance of improvement, even if only temporarily is good. And each new therapy that is developed offers even more hope.

GASTROINTESTINAL CANCER

The intestinal tract is prone to various kinds of tumors, many of which are malignant. Some tumors grow and spread slowly and cause a bowel blockage. Others may be silent until they spread to other parts of the body, which often makes successful treatment difficult. In general, the symptoms include poor appetite, weight loss, bleeding from the bowel, nausea, vomiting, and a change in bowel habits. Often the symptoms are vague, and it may take a long time to discover the tumor. All the factors involved in the causes of gastrointestinal cancer are undetermined. Some families appear to have a tendency to tumors of the bowel, some of which eventually become malignant. People who have had *ulcerative colitis* (an inflammation of the colon and rectum) for many years appear to be more prone to large-bowel cancer than others.

Many claims have been made about dietary influences on intestinal malignancy. Some researchers believe that the small amount of roughage in Western diets is a major factor in the increased incidence of these tumors. Some claim that the large amounts of *nitrosamines* used in processed meats (bacon, salami, bologna, etc.) is responsible. And there are many reports attesting to the belief that large doses of vitamin C or vitamin E will decrease the likelihood of this cancer.

None of these assertions has been proven. A number of on-going studies are trying to determine the relationships between diet, vitamins, and intestinal malignancy, but it will take some years before the results are available. In the meanwhile, it would probably be prudent to increase the amount of fiber in your diet and decrease the amount of processed meats, which, in addition to nitrosamines, contain large amounts of salt. However, there is not enough evidence to merit the use of large doses of vitamin C or vitamin E.

STOMACH CANCER

Cancer of the stomach often gives symptoms of decreased appetite, vomiting, abdominal pain, and anemia, symptoms similar to those of an ulcer. However, the abnormalities do not respond easily to the kinds of treatment that improve ulcer disease. There may be weight loss and uncontrollable vomiting. The diagnosis is usually made with a *barium swallow* and confirmed through a *gastroscopy*.

The treatment is primarily surgical, to remove the diseased stomach and see if the cancer has spread to the abdomen and liver. If the tumor cannot be removed, a bypass operation can be done. Until a few years ago the expectations for survival were poor. However, recent advances in chemotherapy have improved the odds. Many older people have had good responses to chemotherapy after surgery.

INTESTINAL CANCER

Intestinal cancer usually affects the large bowel. It is very uncommon for the small intestine to be affected by malignant disease. The most common symptom leading to discovery of this malignancy is anemia, which shows itself by generalized weakness, or bleeding that may be noticed during a bowel movement. In some instances the first signs of the disease are a change of bowel habits or an actual blockage of the large intestine.

The mainstay of treatment of intestinal cancer is surgery. It is important to remove the tumor to prevent blockage of the bowel and see if the disease has spread. This can be partially established through scans and X-rays prior to surgery. After the operation some people require a *colostomy*, although many have their bowel returned to normal function. Chemotherapy and in some instances radiation therapy may be of value. In the very elderly or the severely debilitated who have tumors of the lower part of the large bowel (rectum), radiotherapy alone can be effective in decreasing symptoms and avoiding the risk of blockage. The results of treatment for cancer of the large bowel can be very satisfying. I have known many older individuals who have lived for many years after having undergone surgery and treatment for this type of malignancy.

CANCER OF THE PANCREAS

Cancer of the pancreas can be painless during the early stages, but the effects can be serious even when the tumor is small. Often, the early symptoms are nonspecific and do not point to the pancreas at all, so a diagnosis may not be made. For unexplained reasons, psychological effects such as depression occur frequently in this disorder. But, since depression is often attributed to the process of aging, tests to discover this tumor may not be done immediately. Weight loss without explanation or a blockage of the bile ducts (connection between the liver and small bowel), causing jaundice, may be the first signs of pancreatic cancer.

Even though X-rays, nuclear scans, and newer methods such as echograms and CAT scans may be done, the diagnosis can still be difficult to establish. I have seen a few older people who were losing weight and feeling depressed undergo repeated X-rays and echograms. When a tumor was not found, treatment was directed to the psychological symptoms, with little improvement. Many months later, symptoms finally appeared or the tumor became large enough for the X-ray or echogram to verify its existence.

If the tumor is found very early, surgery can be successful, but in most cases it is not discovered in time for surgery to be of use. However, surgery can be done to alleviate the symptoms of vomiting and jaundice. If the tumor is blocking the bile ducts, stomach or small intestine, the surgeon can perform a bypass operation to redirect the passage of food and bile around the tumor and delay these symptoms.

There has been a recent nonsurgical advance that allows a temporary improvement in the symptoms caused by jaundice due to blockage of the bile ducts. A thin plastic tube is inserted through the skin into the liver and then directed to pass through the biliary ducts, past the pancreatic cancer and into the duodenum. The procedure can be done under local anesthetic and often allows relief of the itching, nausea, and drowsiness caused by the jaundice.

Frequently, such operations or procedures allow months of comfort that otherwise would not be possible. It would be a mistake to say that the operation is not successful because it does not cure the disease. The relief of symptoms and giving a period of comfort are of great importance and should be attempted whenever pancreatic cancer is diagnosed.

LIVER CANCER

Cancer of the liver unfortunately is common. It can arise in the liver itself, especially in people who suffer from *cirrhosis* as a result of alcohol abuse. Most often, however, it has spread from another source, usually within the abdomen. This is referred to as *metastatic carcinoma* of the liver. In most instances, if cancer has spread to the liver, it usually means the disease is quite advanced, and treatment is directed to give comfort and relieve pain. Chemotherapy so far has had only a limited effect, although certain forms of cancer may respond better than others. Each situation is different. Even though there is no treatment to significantly increase the life span, medications can improve symptoms and decrease discomfort.

CANCER OF THE PROSTATE, BLADDER, AND KIDNEYS

Small nodules of cancer are often inadvertently found in prostate glands removed during the treatment of benign enlargement. It appears that these tiny nodules grow slowly, especially in the very elderly. They may eventually spread locally and then to other parts of the body, particularly to the bones, where prostate cancer can cause a great deal of pain and sometimes spontaneous fractures.

When found early, surgery to remove a malignant growth is possible. Frequently, when the prostate is removed for another reason, any malignancy found by chance can be cured. There may already be evidence of local spread of the disease at the time of diagnosis. Some physicians recommend radiation therapy to the prostate, to cure the disease or decrease its spread at this stage. This is sometimes successful. In many cases, even if the malignant cells have spread to other organs, including the bones, there can be a dramatic and successful response to the surgical removal of the testicles or to hormonal therapy (female hormones). Radiation of the affected bones also is sometimes beneficial in reducing pain.

Many elderly men respond to treatment for long periods of time. With the newer, more potent hormonal medications there can be some swelling of the breasts, but this usually is not unduly uncomfortable. Other forms of chemotherapy may be necessary if removal of the testicles or hormonal therapy have not been effective.

Cancer of the bladder can vary in its degree of malignancy. It usually presents itself as blood in the urine, and this requires immediate medical attention. I have seen people who noticed bleeding one day and because it stopped by itself did not seek medical advice until the tumor had spread.

In the early stages bladder cancer can be diagnosed by *cystoscopy*, and in many instances the tumor can be removed by "burning" it through the cystoscope. Although it may grow again, it can be removed in this fashion on a number of occasions. Less commonly, the tumor can spread quickly, and some physicians recommend radiation therapy with or without surgery to remove the bladder altogether. A replacement bladder can be made from a piece of intestine. Chemotherapy can decrease the spread of the disease to other parts of the body and improve the symptoms.

The kidneys can harbor a malignant growth for quite awhile before it reveals itself. It, too, may first show its presence as blood in the urine. Some people suffer from unexplainable weight loss and fever before the tumor is found. At times, it is discovered because of a swelling in the abdomen or the legs.

Diagnosis usually requires a kidney X-ray (IVP), and at early stages, an echogram and CAT scan can provide a diagnosis. Treatment usually includes surgery to remove the kidney. Some hormonal drugs can decrease the progress of this disease and afford some improvement in symptoms if it should return after surgery.

GYNECOLOGICAL TUMORS

The most common gynecological tumors are found in the cervix (the part of the uterus that projects into the vagina), but growths in the uterus are also common. There has been some controversy about the factors that contribute to the high incidence of such tumors. It appears that women who have had numerous pregnancies may be more prone to cervical cancer.

Cancer of the uterus appears to be somewhat more common in women who take female hormone (estrogen) medications after menopause, even though there are many positive aspects too. The data is conflicting, but it seems that the use of estrogen medications alone increases the chances of developing uterine cancer. If a small amount of *progesterone* is added to the estrogen, the risk seems to decrease a great deal. But the controversy continues as to whether women should take these medications.

Having a Pap test of the cervix every one or two years is an important way to decrease the chance of developing cancer of the cervix or uterus. The Pap smear can pick up the disease in the early stages, when treatment is simpler. If a malignancy is found, local surgical removal of a small part of the cervix or the use of radiation, and recently the use of locally applied chemotherapeutic agents, may be of value. In more advanced stages removal of the whole uterus *(hysterectomy)* may be required. The results are usually good, especially if the disease is found early. Even in advanced cases some improvement in symptoms and relief of discomfort can result from a combination of chemotherapy and radiation therapy.

Cancer of the uterus may first show itself with bleeding after menopause, an important symptom that should never be overlooked. If you have been taking estrogen hormones alone for menopausal symptoms, bleeding during therapy or between cycles of drugs should not occur. Sometimes if progesterone is added to the estrogen, there may be some bleeding between drug cycles. However, if you have never experienced bleeding on these medications you should not develop it at a later date. Do not assume that the symptom is due to hormone therapy. Bleeding of any type should always be reported to your physician.

The ovaries can also be affected by cancer, and growths are

sometimes found during routine gynecological examinations. For this reason, it is important to have a pelvic examination every year or two even after you have stopped menstruating. The first symptom may be a feeling of fullness in the lower part of the abdomen.

Treatment includes surgery to remove the tumor, and some women require radiation therapy or chemotherapy. The response to treatment is usually good. Although the tumor may return, a further course of treatment can be started, and is often effective.

BRAIN TUMORS

Because the brain is surrounded by bone, there is very little room for a tumor to grow without increasing the pressure within the skull. Therefore, the symptoms of brain tumors occur fairly early, when the growths are still small. Some brain tumors start within the brain itself and cause their damage by enlarging quickly, rather than spreading to other organs. Others have spread from another part of the body, and sometimes the first sign of the initial cancer is the brain tumor.

Not all tumors of the brain are malignant. One common type of benign tumor found in older people is a *meningioma*. These grow very slowly but gradually cause memory lapses, changes in personality or weakness of a limb. Often, they can be safely and successfully removed.

Malignant tumors of the brain, however, are difficult to treat. The first symptoms may likewise be a change in personality, impairment of memory and judgment, agitation, or even depression. In the early stages the diagnosis may waver between an emotional disorder and a disease of the nervous system. The early tests, which may include a nuclear brain scan and CAT scan, as well as an electroencephalogram (EEG), may be inconclusive. The progress of the illness is usually fast, and ultimately there may be numbness or tingling, weakness in a limb, or vision impairment. On some occasions a seizure (fit), as might be seen in epilepsy, can occur.

If the tumor is near the surface of the brain, an attempt is made to remove it surgically. Radiation therapy and *cortisone* medication often decrease brain swelling and pressure, thus temporarily improving symptoms. The illness eventually progresses, however, and patients ultimately slip into a deep coma.

BONE CANCER

Malignant tumors originating in the bones are rare in the elderly. However, malignant growths from other parts of the body frequently spread to the bones. The usual symptoms are those of pain and pressure. If the bone becomes weakened by the growth, it can fracture spontaneously, often without a fall or trauma. Because it is difficult to understand how a bone can be fractured without a fall, I have seen nurses unnecessarily accused of being rough with older patients and causing a bone to break, when in fact it was the result of a cancerous growth.

Some kinds of malignant growths that spread to the bones respond very well to treatment. For example, cancer of the prostate with severe spread to the bones will improve or give no symptoms for many years after testicle removal or with the use of hormone therapy. Radiation therapy can relieve the bone pain quickly and effectively, even though it will not cure the cancer. A broken bone may have to be surgically repaired and then treated with radiation. This combination of treatment can prevent the patient from becoming completely disabled by the fracture.

CANCER OF THE LYMPH NODES

The lymph nodes, found throughout the body, are often referred to as the "glands" that in childhood become swollen or painful during an infection. They are part of the normal defense mechanism of the body. The spleen serves a similar purpose and is frequently involved in the same disorders as the lymph nodes. The lymph nodes and spleen produce special cells (an important one being lymphocytes) that manufacture antibodies and help combat infection.

Cancer of the lymph nodes and spleen is called *lymphoma,* and there are many varieties. The symptoms depend on which lymph nodes have become enlarged. The disease can begin as a lump in the neck or groin. Tumors that expand within the abdomen may not be felt, but there may be an unusual degree of fatigue, and at times the temperature may become intermittently elevated, without any sign of infection. It is not uncommon for afflicted individuals to receive a few courses of different antibiotics to treat a fever that does not stay down despite such therapy. Some people become anemic, whereas others become more susceptible to infections which may complicate the appearance of the fever.

To make an accurate diagnosis, the physician will usually do a biopsy of a lymph node and perhaps take a bone marrow specimen, a liver biopsy, X-rays, and scans to determine how far the disease has spread. Depending on the extent of the disease, treatment consists of radiation therapy alone or with *combination chemotherapy.* The response to treatment can be remarkable. If the disease is limited to one area, it may be cured. Even in those who have evidence of the disease in many parts of the body, the illness can be halted for months or years. In addition, so many new drugs are becoming available that even if the ailment returns there is a good chance that new medications will be effective. Treatment should never be denied because of age alone.

LEUKEMIA AND MULTIPLE MYELOMA

Normally, there are different kinds of white cells in the body, including *polymorphonuclear white cells, lymphocytes* and *plasma cells*. They have different appearances and serve different purposes which, however, are related. Their main function is to help combat infection. They do this by various methods, such as making antibodies that help destroy harmful bacteria or removing them from the circulation by ingesting them. A malignant growth of white cells is called *leukemia*.

The types of leukemia that affect the elderly are *chronic leukemias*, which progress much more slowly than those that occur in younger individuals. Each type of leukemia arises from one kind of white blood cell, either polymorphonuclear or lymphocyte. Because of its slow progress, patients can have leukemia for many years without problems. The symptoms include a decreased defense against infection and some weakness because of anemia. Sometimes the spleen, liver and lymph nodes may enlarge, and bones can become painful as the illness advances. There is often a tendency to bruise and bleed easily.

Treatment is usually not necessary during early stages, but a number of medications and, occasionally, radiation therapy can successfully slow the progress of the disease later on. If the spleen becomes too enlarged and painful, it may have to be removed. After many years, the disease suddenly may progress rapidly. Although at this stage it may be difficult to treat, some forms of chemotherapy are sometimes effective.

An unusual disease of the white cells is caused by the development of a malignant growth of plasma cells. The disease, *multiple myeloma*, produces abnormal proteins which, although similar to antibodies, do not have the ability to combat infection. In fact, these abnormal antibodies interfere with the normal defense mechanism and make the person more susceptible to harmful bacteria.

The symptoms include anemia, weight loss and, quite frequently, bone pain. Sometimes the abnormal protein in the blood causes a blockage of blood vessels. The diagnosis usually requires a bone marrow biopsy, in addition to blood tests. There are various forms of therapy for this illness. It will often respond to treatment for a few years and further improvement is possible with some of the newer drugs.

Whatever the form of cancer, treatment is available to decrease its spread, relieve the symptoms, and in early stages perhaps cure it altogether. And newer therapies are being discovered. It is important that you know what treatments will be used and what their possible effects will be, both negative and positive. Sometimes there is nothing more to be done, but even in the most desperate situation, it should be possible to improve the symptoms and relieve discomfort. Do not be afraid to express your fears to your physician: Tell him what you are feeling and how you would like him to help.

CHAPTER 15

Neurological (Nervous System) Disorders

The nervous system is made up of the *brain*, *spinal cord*, and *nerves*. The brain and spinal cord are protected from injury by the surrounding bones of the skull and vertebral column (spine). Nerves leave the spinal cord and make their way through small outlet holes in the vertebral column to supply the muscles and organs.

Motor nerves bring impulses, or messages, *from* the brain and spinal cord to the body. *Sensory nerves* go from the body *back to* the spinal cord and brain and convey messages. The motor and sensory nerves sometimes travel together for part of their journey through the body but usually divide when they enter the spinal cord and brain. The brain and spinal cord contain nerve cells that interconnect with each other and send messages to different parts of the nervous system. Unfortunately, they cannot repair themselves once they have been severely damaged. However, some can be lost without significant impairment of function. If many are damaged at the same time, there will usually be some permanent interference in the

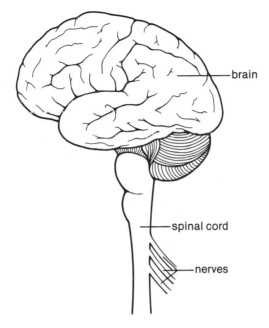

NERVOUS SYSTEM.

working of that part of the nervous system. If the blood supply to the brain and spinal cord is disrupted, there can be serious damage to the nervous system.

Older people are more prone to suffer from diseases of their nervous system. These illnesses account for a large number of the older individuals who require institutionalization. For many people, nervous system disease is the greatest fear. Numerous patients have told me that they would rather die than be institutionalized with a severe, incapacitating disorder.

STROKES

We are all terrified of losing our mental and physical independence, and a stroke is probably the most frightening event

319

of all. Strokes are more common in older people, and their effects can be devastating. However, a great deal can be done to decrease the risk of strokes and improve the outcome.

Stroke means the *sudden*, spontaneous loss of use, feeling, or control of one or more limbs or the impairment of speech and mental function. It may also be complicated by problems with balance and vision. In order for such an episode to be called a stroke, it must occur suddenly. Similar nervous system impairment can happen more slowly and be the result of other diseases, such as a brain tumor or abscess.

The most common cause of strokes is damage to the blood vessels supplying the brain. Many individuals develop athero-sclerosis, and they are more likely to experience brain damage from one of these blood vessels leaking or becoming blocked by a blood clot that forms on the uneven surface of the diseased artery.

A stroke can occur when small particles of a blood clot become dislodged from a diseased heart and travel to the brain. This results in a *cerebral embolus*, and it is more com-mon in older people because heart disease is more prevalent. Many people suffer from high blood pressure, which left un-treated can weaken the blood vessels in the brain. A stroke occurs when one of these vessels bursts.

A stroke can vary in its appearance, severity, and duration. Some people suffer from a weakness of a limb or speech impairment for a few minutes or hours and then the symptoms improve. Others may feel numbness and tingling of their face or hands, which also passes in time. These attacks are often called *transient strokes* because the symptoms improve spon-taneously.

A stroke that occurs, returns again, and wanes once more may be the signal of a severe episode that will become perma-nent. This signal should be reported to your physician im-mediately.

Sometimes the first episode of nervous system disease may be a stroke that does not improve within minutes or hours. This is often referred to as a *completed stroke*, and the damage is not reversible because the brain, when injured severely by an interruption of blood supply, cannot retrieve its function. The symptoms may be a loss of speech and consciousness, as well as weakness of one side of the body.

During the first few hours and days after a completed stroke has occurred, the individual may not be able to respond to normal environmental stimulation. The level of consciousness may be impaired. It is during this crucial period that complications such as pneumonia and problems with heart ailments set in. However, with careful observation and treatment most people can be brought through this period and undertake a program of rehabilitation.

One condition that occurs in elderly individuals can mimic a stroke, but if found and treated early can have a more positive outcome. This is called a *subdural hematoma* and is the result of bleeding within the skull, between the lining of the brain and the bones that surround it. It can occur following a fall, especially if the person is taking anticoagulants (blood thinners). Sometimes it occurs without injury, and the symptoms may develop gradually, with an eventual weakness of limbs, loss of balance, and changes in personality, speech, and memory. If the blood clot (hematoma) is removed through surgery, the results can be dramatic. This type of surgery is so simple that it should never be refused because of age.

Can strokes be prevented?

The main factors responsible for strokes include high blood pressure and *atherosclerosis*. As of yet, we do not know completely how to prevent atherosclerosis, although some evidence suggests that changes in the diet, with a decrease in the amount of animal fat, may play a role. However, no one can say that if you stop eating animal fats altogether you will not suffer from strokes. This may be partially true for younger people, but it has not yet been proven.

The reduction of high blood pressure, however, has definitely been shown to decrease the likelihood of a stroke. Anticoagulants have been found to decrease the likelihood of strokes in certain people. Unfortunately, some of these medications may have serious side effects and are used only in certain situations. If you have shown evidence of a transient stroke, your physician may use anticoagulants to try to prevent another stroke. Anticoagulation therapy must be carefully supervised to avoid the risks of bleeding.

Recent evidence indicates that medications such as aspirin and other drugs that affect platelets can decrease the stickiness of the blood and prevent strokes in certain individuals. Some physicians therefore prescribe small doses of *aspirin, dipyridamole,* and *sulfinpyrazone* for potential stroke victims. It will take more time and research before it is known for certain whether these platelet-inhibiting drugs are effective. Their risk, however, is less than with anticoagulants.

Under certain circumstances surgery may prevent a stroke. If you have a partial blockage of one of the main arteries going to the brain, this can be corrected. An *angiogram* of these blood vessels is necessary in order to make the diagnosis.

How are strokes treated?

If part of the brain is permanently damaged by a stroke, that part will no longer function. However, the rest of the brain continues to operate. At the time of a stroke, one may be at risk of developing pneumonia, so hospitalization is usually required. If the stroke is mild, this may not be necessary. A stroke victim is sometimes placed in a special Intensive Care Unit to prevent complications. Often this is not necessary.

The rest of the treatment is directed to prevent further brain damage and to teach the remaining healthy brain some of the tasks that were previously done by the damaged part. Therefore, although no treatment can reverse the damage, a great deal can be done to improve the outcome.

REHABILITATION

The term *rehabilitation*, or physical therapy, means those types of therapy that will help you reach the maximum degree of function after an illness or injury. Following a stroke, the main difficulties are usually those of walking and balance, the use of arms and hands, and speech.

Some people feel that if a person receives enough physical therapy following a stroke he will eventually retrieve all impaired faculties. This often leads to frustration because the patient and family expected greater improvement than might be possible. Rehabilitation teaches you how to use other parts of the brain, as well as other nerves and muscles, to take over the tasks of the damaged area. The goal is to achieve the most normal function possible, which may not be a full return of abilities.

Who is responsible for rehabilitation?

The specialty is called *physiatry*, and as in other medical specialties, a physiatrist has a basic training in all aspects of medicine with a special interest in rehabilitation after neurological, muscular, and bone diseases.

Working with the physiatrist is the paramedical staff—physiotherapists, occupational therapists, and speech therapists. Many medical centers are well equipped and specifically committed to treating older patients.

Will more rehabilitation therapy
result in more improvement?

If one has suffered from damage to the brain, nerves, bones, or muscles, there is a good chance of improvement. There is, however, a limit to the benefits that can be expected, especially following severe brain damage. Most therapists can anticipate what degree of improvement might be expected and how long it will take to reach the utmost level of function. In the older person it can take longer.

Once it is determined that further therapy will not result in additional improvement, you will receive instruction on how to maintain optimal function on your own. This is very important. It is a shame to lose the advantages of a rehabilitation program once it is finished for lack of a well-outlined maintenance program.

What treatments and aids can be expected in a rehabilitation program?

The types of treatment and aids are many. Therapists teach special exercises to improve body function and frequently use mechanical aids, including walkers and canes. Treatment with heat, ultrasound, and possibly cortisone injections into painful joints may be required. Exercises in a warm pool under supervision may be valuable. Splints may be used to relieve pain. There are special devices to help you to dress and to use the bathroom and kitchen, thus assisting you to become independent.

If you suffer from a neurological disease and want to return home, a consultation and home visit with a rehabilitation expert should be arranged. Your home will be examined and changes made, possibly including handrails on walls or near the toilet or tub to help you get up with the least difficulty. Your kitchen may be altered so that the sink, refrigerator, and stove can be used easily and safely. In most cases the degree and cost of alterations are relatively small. And they may make the difference between being able to return home to function relatively independently, or requiring permanent institutionalization.

PARKINSON'S DISEASE

Parkinson's disease is more common in the elderly. Because the degree of symptoms vary, some people may be completely incapacitated by the illness, whereas others may not even realize that they have it. The most prominent symptoms are slowness in walking, shaking and stiffness of the limbs, and difficulty in speaking and swallowing. Your facial muscles may droop and friends or family may wonder why you always appear "unhappy." You may develop a "shuffling gait," which means that you do not lift your legs from the floor when you walk and often you have difficulty in turning. This often causes falls. The difficulty you experience in walking and getting out of a chair or bed may be attributed to arthritis or "just growing old." Often, because the symptoms are mild, a diagnosis may be over-looked. Tranquilizers or drugs for the treatment of a hiatus hernia can cause a drug-induced type of Parkinson's disease.

How is Parkinson's disease diagnosed?

Your physician should be aware that some medications pre-cipitate or aggravate Parkinson's disease. A careful history and physical examination is usually required to confirm the diag-nosis. Your physician should watch you walk, turn, and get out of a chair. He should also feel the way your arms move as he pushes them back and forth. With Parkinson's disease, he can feel that the muscles are intermittently stiff when they are moved. This is usually sufficient to make a diagnosis. There is no laboratory test to diagnose this illness.

Is there memory loss in Parkinson's disease?

Even though some people with severe Parkinson's disease have difficulty speaking, their memory and judgment are usually quite good. There is some suggestion that if the disease goes on for many years some loss of mental function may occur, but this is usually not as severe as in other diseases of the brain. Unfortunately, many people assume that because a person cannot move or speak quickly the mind is also impaired, and this can be very frustrating and aggravating.

Is treatment effective?

During the past few years major advances in the treatment of Parkinson's disease have been made. With the newer medications, such as L-Dopa or levodopa-carbidopa, most people can expect a marked improvement in their function. Other effective medications, taken alone or in combination, can also be prescribed. If your illness is not recognized and treated, you might become bedridden. This is a great shame when a few tablets a day might allow you to walk again.

For example, recently I saw an elderly immigrant from the Soviet Union. She had experienced difficulty in walking for many years and was told that it was because of her age. At one point, while abroad, she fell and fractured her hip. Surgery was not done because she was considered "too old" and "could not walk anyway." She was allowed to leave the Soviet Union and accompanied her daughter to Canada.

She had severe Parkinson's disease and showed an excellent improvement after being treated with medications. Even with the poorly healed hip, she was able to walk with the assistance of a walker by the time she was discharged from the hospital.

Are there any dangers in treatment?

Some people may not be able to tolerate the newer drugs, which can cause agitation and nightmares. There may also be a lowering of blood pressure or abnormal heart rhythms. A few patients are so sensitive that very small doses can cause involuntary shaking movements. These, however, usually do not interfere with walking and are often preferable to the stiffness that occurs when the medication is discontinued.

If you cannot tolerate the medication, it should be stopped, then started again in a smaller dose, and increased very gradually. Sometimes a different drug can be substituted. Fortunately, there are very few people with Parkinson's disease who cannot tolerate any of the medications at all.

After many years of drug therapy, the disease may become uncontrollable. However, new drugs are always being tested that may improve the symptoms that no longer respond to the existing medications. Whenever a new drug becomes available, those people with the most severe symptoms are the first to be treated with it. Stopping the drugs temporarily *(drug holiday)* and then resuming them may lead to improvement.

SENILE TREMOR

One of the more common causes of a *tremor* (shake) that may interfere only minimally with your functioning is *senile tremor*. This is in fact an inaccurate term because the condition often runs in families and can start at any age. It does not mean that there is anything terribly wrong with the nervous system. However, the nuisance and self-consciousness can be intolerable.

Sometimes the *cerebellum*, a part of the brain, becomes impaired, especially if you have been a heavy alcohol drinker. This can lead to an unsteadiness in walking, as well as severe shaking of the hands.

Recently, it has been found that *propranolol*, which is used extensively for angina pectoris and hypertension, can be effective in stopping the shaking of senile tremor. Many people can be helped by this medication, which often works in small doses. However, a few individuals may not respond to its effects.

I saw one man after he had surgery for a broken leg because the surgeon had noticed a tremor. The patient admitted that he had a problem with shaking for many years and that it greatly interfered with his life. He had been a senior executive and for years had tried to avoid large company meetings because of his disability. He had a typical familial tremor and was treated with small doses of propranolol. The next time I saw him, he said, "If I knew that all I had to do to get rid of this shaking was to fall and break my leg and get put on these pills, I would have jumped out of a window years ago."

MOTOR NEURONE DISEASE

Motor neurone disease, which affects the nerves and muscles, is more often found in younger people, but it may start in the later years. The first symptoms are usually muscular weakness, twitching, and clumsiness. Within a short period there may be difficulty in speaking, swallowing, and breathing. There is a tendency to inhale food and saliva and develop *aspiration pneumonia.*

So far no treatment has been found to correct this illness. Toward the end of the disease extensive nursing care is necessary, so hospitalization is often required. In some, the illness progresses slowly. Unfortunately, most older people die from the disease within two or three years.

MYASTHENIA GRAVIS

Myasthenia gravis, a disorder in which the nerves going to muscles do not transmit the impulses properly, results in weakness of the muscles in the arms and legs. The disease may begin very gradually and take many months before the disability is severe enough for you to seek help. One of the first symptoms can be eye weakness, with difficulty in focusing and double vision from time to time. You may develop difficulty in speaking. The amount of weakness may vary from day to day and at different times during the day. Swallowing may become impaired, and you may have difficulty clearing the saliva from your throat.

An *electromyelogram* and *nerve conduction studies* can help diagnose this disorder. Certain drugs which temporarily reverse the abnormality can be used to verify the diagnosis. Some people respond well to medications that improve the electrical impulses at the connection between the nerves and muscles; other individuals respond to cortisone treatment. It may be necessary to remove the remnants of the *thymus gland*, which sits behind the breastbone. Although this operation can be difficult, it frequently results in major relief of the symptoms, even though drugs may still be required for its control. Before surgery, some medical centers first treat patients with a blood exchange to clear the body of the substances that aggravate the disease. This temporarily improves the condition until surgery can be done. Not all medical centers are equipped for all aspects of therapy. A neurologist can direct you to the most suitable medical center in your vicinity.

Several other disorders can affect the muscles and nerves and cause weakness and pain, or both. Some illnesses occur with inflammatory conditions such as arthritis, whereas others result from virus infections or malignant disorders. At times it can be difficult to unravel the cause of muscle weakness and a *muscle biopsy* and special *electrical studies* are necessary. Some of these peculiar ailments are treatable, whereas others will improve or deteriorate depending on the nature of the underlying disorder.

CHAPTER 16

Eye, Ear, Nose and Throat Disorders

THE EYE

Light enters the eye through the *cornea*, which is located at the very front of the eye and is completely transparent. It then passes through the *pupil*, which is the black center of the eye. This in fact is the aperture in the *iris*, which gives eyes their color. The iris can open and close, thereby causing the size of the pupil to change. By varying the size of the opening, the amount of light entering the eye can be controlled. If the light is very bright, the pupil is small and, when it is dark, the pupil is wide open.

After light passes through the pupil, it is focused by the *lens*, which sits behind the iris. The focused light rays are directed to the *retina*, which is located at the back of the eye and contains special cells that translate the light images into nervous messages. These are carried by the *optic nerves* from the retina to the brain, where they are interpreted.

Illness can affect one or many parts of the eye. Some

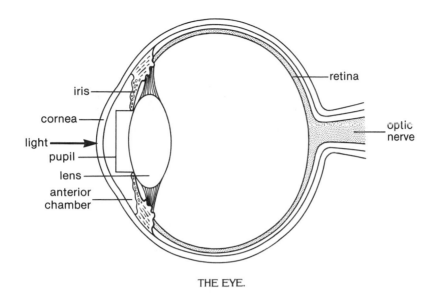

iris

cornea

light

pupil

lens

anterior
chamber

retina

optic
nerve

THE EYE.

problems, such as infection, affect people at any age, whereas others are more likely to occur as you grow older. In the older person a decrease or loss of vision can be devastating because it interferes with feelings of self-worth and exaggerates the effects of isolation, dependency, and loneliness. If you are not able to read or watch television, you may become cut off from the everyday activities of the world.

You should have a thorough periodic examination by a physician or *ophthalmologist* to ensure that your vision has not deteriorated as the result of disease. Any sudden change in vision should be checked immediately, because many illnesses that cause blindness can be prevented or treated.

CATARACTS

A *cataract* is a condition in which the lens of the eye becomes opaque, which means vision is impaired because light cannot pass through. Many older people develop cataracts, and the exact cause is not clear. In the early stages there may be some haziness and decrease in vision, but you may still be able to see adequately. An ophthalmologist will usually recommend removal of a cataract only when the vision in both eyes becomes greatly impaired. He will remove the cataract from one eye first, and if this goes well, he may or may not operate on the second eye some months later. Not everyone requires *binocular* (two-eyed) vision, and for many a surgical procedure to restore vision in one eye is sufficient.

Can a cataract be removed under a local anesthetic?

The type of anesthetic depends on the surgical technique and your ability to cooperate during surgery if a local anesthetic is used. In some situations a local anesthetic is preferred, whereas in others a general anesthetic may be safer. The decision is made by the physician, surgeon, and anesthetist before surgery. A local anesthetic reduces the likelihood of anesthetic complications and decreases your period of convalescence.

What is best—a lens implant during surgery, or contact lenses or glasses after surgery?

The greatest experience has been with glasses after a cataract removal, although there are disadvantages. You will have a narrow range of vision, and if you misplace or lose your glasses your vision will be poor. Details cannot be distinguished without glasses, and you will see only light and movement.

Contact lenses avoid some of these problems, but they are often difficult to insert as you grow older, particularly if you have arthritis or a shaking of the hands. If they can be used, they are very effective and, in some people, they are preferable to glasses.

The newer technique of *lens implant* has many advantages over glasses and contact lenses. The lens usually can be implanted with relatively few complications. Vision improves enormously and often is very close to normal. And you will see well immediately *after* surgery.

What are the dangers of cataract surgery?

Your eye doctor will try to determine the likelihood of your vision improving with cataract surgery. Unfortunately, the retina may be so damaged that surgery does not improve your vision. Although this happens rarely, it can be very upsetting after you have placed so much hope on the surgery.

After surgery, infection, bleeding, retinal detachment, or a blockage of a blood vessel to the eye can occur. These complications cannot be predicted, and rarely can they be prevented. However, they are quite unusual, and vision can usually be restored despite complications.

GLAUCOMA

Glaucoma is the result of an increase in pressure within the eye. As the pressure builds, the retina is slowly damaged and eventually destroyed. You may have *chronic glaucoma* without any symptoms until your vision becomes severely damaged. You may notice a distortion of vision and halos around lights or find that your vision has become poor. During an attack of *acute glaucoma*, there may be sudden eye pain, redness, and a rapid deterioration of vision. In most people, however, the disease is not painful, but it can progress slowly and insidiously, leading to impaired vision or blindness.

You should have your eyes checked at least once a year. The eye pressure should be measured to determine whether it is elevated. This can be done by a family doctor who has experience in the technique or by an ophthalmologist. It may not be sufficient to have your vision tested by an optometrist, and in some areas, optometrists are not trained or allowed to measure eye pressure. Glaucoma might not be diagnosed when your vision is being checked for glasses by an optometrist. Ask whether he has measured your eye pressure when you visit him.

Some medications used to treat depression, heart disease, or bowel disorders can increase the risk of glaucoma. Some eye drops can also make glaucoma worse. If you suffer from glaucoma, ask your physician about the effects of new drugs on this condition. And make sure that any physician you see knows that you have glaucoma.

What is the treatment for glaucoma?

The most important part of treatment is early diagnosis. When high eye pressure is found before there is severe damage to vision, most people can be treated successfully with eyedrops or medications that decrease the pressure. If the eye drops are not completely effective, surgery may be recommended. During an attack of acute glaucoma, you will first receive intensive medical treatment to decrease the pressure. This may be followed by surgery to allow the excess fluid to drain from the eye. In most instances glaucoma can be treated and controlled if the diagnosis is made early. It would be tragic to lose your vision from a condition that can be so effectively treated, so have your vision and eye pressure tested at least once a year.

OTHER EYE DISORDERS

What is a retinal detachment?

The retina contains the cells and nerves that translate light into images. If the retina becomes detached, you may feel as if a curtain is covering your eye, or you may experience flashing lights. Your vision will become blurred, and if untreated, you could lose it altogether. A retinal detachment can occur for no apparent reason, or it may result from an injury or a complication of other eye surgery, such as that for cataracts. It is more likely to occur if you are severely *myopic* (nearsighted) or have diabetes mellitus with eye complications.

Is there any treatment for a retinal detachment?

It is now possible for the retina to be reattached to the back of your eye. The earlier the surgery is done, the better the chance of success. An eye surgeon can "glue" the retina in place, and in many instances vision will be effectively restored.

What is macular degeneration?

This disorder affects older people. The central part of the retina, the *macula*, which is responsible for reading and seeing small objects, gradually becomes damaged. It can occur in both eyes simultaneously. You may have difficulty seeing fine details, and you will notice that changing your glasses offers no improvement.

The diagnosis requires a special examination by an ophthalmologist. Although the disorder cannot be treated, magnifying glasses and other visual aids can partially improve your vision.

Why do elderly people with diabetes mellitus have vision problems?

A diabetic who requires insulin is more prone to develop severe eye disease. It usually occurs in those who have suffered from diabetes for long periods (twenty or twenty-five years). You may find that your vision has gradually or suddenly decreased. Sometimes the blood vessels in the eye become weakened and bleed, or they expand abnormally and interfere with vision. You may notice a clouding and blurring that may suddenly become worse. This usually means a hemorrhage has occurred within your eye, or your retina has become detached as a complication of the eye disease.

Is there any treatment for diabetic eye disease?

Until recently, the results of treatment were often disappointing and in some instances very dangerous. Some eye doctors now use a *laser beam* to prevent the small blood vessels from bleeding, thus perhaps slowing the disease and keeping it under control. It usually does not cure it, but it forestalls rapid deterioration and blindness. The better the diabetes is controlled, the less rapidly the eye problems will progress.

One major recent advance in the surgery for diabetic eye disease is an operation called a *vitrectomy*. The eye surgeon cuts out and removes the extra blood vessels and blood clots that block vision. It does not always succeed completely in the older person, but it may significantly improve vision. The operation is still relatively new and not performed in all medical centers. It will take a few years before its role in the treatment of this disease can be fully evaluated.

What is a retinal artery occlusion?

The main blood vessel to the eye, the retinal artery, can become blocked by a blood clot or a piece of *atheroma* (fatty material) that comes from a diseased blood vessel. This can result in a sudden, complete or partial loss of vision. Unfortunately, the condition usually cannot be reversed. Some vision may gradually return, depending on the degree of initial damage and whether the main artery or one of its smaller branches was blocked.

What is temporal arteritis?

This is a disease of blood vessels and muscles that can affect vision. It often accompanies the type of rheumatism called *polymyalgia rheumatica*, and it is most common in the elderly. It may occur along with aches and pains in the muscles and joints. You may experience a severe headache and notice a change in your vision.

With an early diagnosis and treatment with cortisone, your vision may be saved and the other symptoms will disappear. Unfortunately, if the diagnosis is not made, the sight in the affected eye may be lost. Cortisone treatment, however, is usually recommended to prevent the second eye from being affected.

THE EAR

Some common problems that can seriously affect your ability to be independent are the result of diseases of the ear. The ear performs two major functions: hearing and balance. The *outer ear* gathers sound and concentrates it through the *ear canal* until it reaches the *ear drum*, the beginning of the *middle ear*. The middle ear is responsible for transmitting the sound through a number of small bones to the *inner ear*. Within the inner ear is a mechanism that translates the sound waves into nerve impulses, which are sent to the brain for interpretation. The important balance apparatus is contained within the inner ear.

Is deafness a natural consequence of aging?

Many people will develop some mild impairment of hearing as they grow older. Often it will not significantly interfere with your function, although in some instances it can be disabling. If you suffered from an injury to your eardrums many years ago and it was not properly treated, a decrease in hearing may persist and become worse with time. This might respond to surgical repair. Wax in the ears does not usually cause a decrease in hearing. However, if your ear canals are completely blocked by wax, you may experience some decrease in your hearing in addition to a feeling of fullness or pressure in the ear. In this case a hearing aid may not work properly, but this improves after the wax is removed.

One cause of decreased hearing is *otosclerosis*. Even though it is more common in younger people, it can progress throughout life. In this condition the small bones in the ear that help

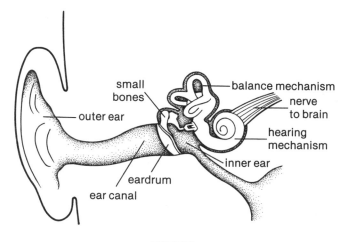

THE EAR.

transmit sound become "stuck" together and no longer vibrate properly, so the sound waves do not pass the middle ear to the inner ear.

There is some controversy as to whether older people might benefit from surgery to make the bones mobile again. There is good evidence that in a few older individuals, this type of surgery may be very successful. In some instances the surgery alone restores hearing. In others surgery can improve the results of using a hearing aid, which may be needed after the operation.

A very common cause of hearing loss is the deterioration of the inner ear *(nerve deafness)*. The exact cause is unknown, but it affects most older people to some degree. Some people seem to be able to hear with no problem until they are very old, whereas others begin to lose their hearing earlier. Although no special treatment will return hearing if you have this problem, some improvements can be made. In some instances a hearing aid may be of value, although it is less often helpful in this kind of deafness.

Aspirin, often prescribed for arthritic conditions, can interfere

338

with hearing and may cause ringing of your ears. This improves when the aspirin is stopped. Some strong antibiotics used in serious infections may also interfere with hearing.

How is hearing tested?

Although you may notice that your hearing has deteriorated, often it is your family and friends who first become aware of it. If the problem has occurred suddenly, urgent medical attention is recommended. Usually the deterioration is gradual and often takes a long time before you recognize the degree of your disability.

To examine the cause of your hearing loss properly, an *audiogram* (hearing test) should be done. This will usually help determine the type of deafness and the most helpful treatment. A full ear examination is usually done in conjunction with the audiogram.

Does everyone with hearing loss benefit from a hearing aid?

A hearing aid will not return hearing to all deaf people. An audiogram is helpful in determining whether your hearing will improve with the use of a hearing aid. Therefore, this test should be done before one is purchased.

The advice of an ear, nose, and throat specialist should be sought before you invest in a hearing aid. A reputable dealer should be contacted by your physician so that the right one is chosen. It is sometimes difficult to know whether you will benefit from a hearing aid or even be able to tolerate one. A "trial" should be arranged with the dealer before it is purchased. Such an expensive piece of equipment should not be bought without a careful evaluation and an acceptable financial arrangement. It is important that a plan be made for proper maintenance of your hearing aid. You and your family should know how to replace batteries and make normal adjustments.

I knew an elderly gentleman with severe deafness who was hospitalized for another problem. The nurses felt that he was probably "senile" because he never answered their questions. His hearing aid had been removed and put on his bedside table at the time of his admission to the hospital. Even after it was put in his ear, he did not seem to improve. When the batteries were changed, he perked up and smiled. His "senility" disappeared immediately!

A hearing impairment also can be ameliorated by various home aids. Telephone amplifying devices allow you to hear more clearly, and radios and televisions can be modified so that you can continue to enjoy these important aspects of modern life.

Can dizziness be caused by ear problems?

A damaged inner ear can cause problems in balance and lead to dizziness. You may recall attacks of dizziness in your younger years resulting from an inflammation of the balance mechanism within the ear. The dizziness that you now suffer from may be a consequence of that damage. In this instance dizziness and loss of balance usually occur when you physically change your position. It may be momentary, as when you stand up from a bed or chair. You should remember to stand up slowly and wait for the dizzy spell to pass before you start walking. This problem is difficult to treat, and most medications have little positive effect. You should learn to anticipate what moves cause your dizziness so that you can avoid them or do them slowly while holding onto something for support.

What causes ringing in the ears?

This may be the result of a simple problem, such as wax in your ears or inflammation, or a more serious consequence of a neurological disease for which there is no treatment. If you take large doses of aspirin for arthritis, you may suffer from ringing in your ears and a decrease in hearing.

You may also experience a "wooshing" in your ears, which can interfere with your sleep and be very upsetting. The cause of this problem is not clear. Sometimes it is the result of blood flowing through a partially narrowed artery in the skull. In most instances it cannot be satisfactorily treated, although small doses of tranquilizers at night may be helpful.

THE NOSE AND THROAT

Problems of the nose and throat are usually less severe in the elderly and may be a continuation of diseases that existed in younger days. Any new problems that arise in later years should be investigated by an *otolaryngologist* (ear, nose, and throat specialist).

What causes hoarseness?

In many instances hoarseness or a deepening of the voice may occur during a cold or flulike illness. In these situations it is short-lived and disappears within a few weeks. You should rest your voice by avoiding loud talking or singing, and use a humidifier if the air in your home is very dry.

If hoarseness lasts for more than two or three weeks, im-mediate medical advice should be sought and your *larynx* (voice box) examined. Tumors, both benign and malignant, can occur on the larynx and cause hoarseness. Malignant tumors, when found in the early stages, can be treated effectively and sometimes cured with radiation. In the later stages surgery may be required.

You might develop hoarseness as part of *hypothyroidism.* The change in your voice may be gradual, and it may be noticed only by friends and family who have not seen you for some time. With proper *thyroid hormone replacement,* your voice should improve.

The habit of constantly clearing the throat can be a nervous quirk related to anxiety and worry or the result of mucus dripping from the back of your nose, in which case treatment with an antihistamine often helps.

What causes dryness of the mouth and nose?

You may suffer from an impairment of the mucus or salivary glands, which normally moisten and lubricate your nose and mouth. Treatment of these disorders is very difficult. You can suck hard candy such as lemon drops to stimulate the salivary glands to produce some fluid. Good oral hygiene is important, including caring for your teeth, drinking plenty of fluids and rinsing your mouth frequently. Rinses with bicarbonate of soda are sometimes helpful.

Some medications cause dryness of the mouth, particularly tranquilizers, sedatives, and medications used for urinary incontinence, some intestinal disorders, high blood pressure, and certain heart conditions. If you take any of these drugs, ask your physician if they might be responsible.

Small amounts of lanolin or petroleum jelly are beneficial in decreasing nose dryness. If the cause is allergy, a small amount of cortisone cream may be helpful. A common aggravating factor is extreme dryness of the air in the home that occurs in the winter when the heat is on. A humidifier can ease the problem considerably.

What causes nose bleeds?

A nose bleed can result from high blood pressure or from an infection such as a cold or flu. Some people "pick" at their noses and cause injury that results in bleeding. Your blood vessels do not close as quickly as in younger people.

If the bleeding is severe, you should apply firm pressure to the sides of your nose by squeezing just above your nostrils for five or ten minutes. If your nose does not stop bleeding, seek emergency medical attention because you can lose a great deal of blood within a very brief period.

CHAPTER 17

Arthritic Conditions

ARTHRITIS AND RHEUMATISM

Arthritis and *rheumatism* describe many different diseases, but the features that they all share are pain, swelling, and interference in the normal movement of either one or more joints. Some kinds of arthritis affect only one joint, whereas others affect many simultaneously. Some are more common in older people, and others are rare in people of all ages. Many older people often assume that their aches and pains are the result of arthritis, and that arthritis is a natural consequence of aging. Both of these assumptions are far from the truth.

The most common type of arthritis in the older individual is *osteoarthritis*, which usually affects one joint at a time, although many joints can gradually become involved. Some studies suggest that this condition affects from 15 to 25 percent of people over the age of 65. Osteoarthritis is caused by a gradual but progressive wearing down of the usually smooth covering (cartilage) of the joint bones. The cause of the destruction is not completely known: In some people it appears to be the result of a previous injury or trauma; in others it appears for no apparent reason. The end result, however, is that the joint surfaces become painful when they move. Often, the large joints that support much of the body's weight become affected first, frequently the hips, knees, and back. Sometimes it affects the smaller joints of the hands and feet. The joint becomes swollen as opposing bones become widened and fluid accumulates. If it is badly damaged, it may not move or support weight properly, and it can interfere with walking or bending. Sometimes a joint that is affected but not uncomfortable may suddenly become swollen and painful as the result of inflammation or infection. This must be treated immediately.

Rheumatoid arthritis occurs less commonly for the first time in the older person, but if you have suffered from this illness during your younger years, it may continue to afflict you as you grow older. This illness can affect many parts of the body simultaneously, in addition to the joints. More than one joint is usually involved, often the smaller joints of the hands, wrists, feet, neck, and jaw. Some people develop fever, loss of appetite, weight loss, and heart and lung problems. The joints, however, are the most obvious and painful focus of the disease.

The course of rheumatoid arthritis varies: Some people contract a severe case in the beginning; for others it may be mild and create little disability. The symptoms may come and go, with severe bouts followed by long periods of comfort, which are again aggravated by episodes of pain and poor health. Unfortunately, self-diagnosis and treatment for arthritic symptoms is common. This can interfere with a proper assessment and a well-designed plan of treatment, which often results in great improvement and relief of symptoms.

Can other types of arthritis affect the older person?

If you suffer from *psoriasis*, you may develop an arthritis that looks similar to rheumatoid arthritis but is less serious. The illness may come and go according to the severity of your skin disease.

Gout, due to an elevation of *uric acid* which deposits in the joints, can occur for the first time in the older person with or without a previous history of gout. You may know that the uric acid level in your blood has been high in the past but never had an attack of gout. You may be taking diuretics or receiving chemotherapy treatment for a malignancy, especially one affecting the blood, which often raises the level of uric acid. In gouty arthritis, usually only one joint is painful at a time, although occasionally more than one joint flares up. It affects the smaller joints, such as the big toe, and the pain is often severe, usually with redness and heat in the area of the inflamed joint.

Pseudogout almost always occurs only in the elderly. The *pseudo* means that it *looks* like gout, although much larger joints, such as the knees and hips, are mainly affected. It is not associated with an elevation of uric acid as is gout. Another irritant, *calcium pyrophosphate*, settles in the joint and causes it to become inflamed. Pseudogout often occurs in a joint that already has osteoarthritis. It can occur after a physical illness that does not appear to be related to the joints, such as a heart attack or infection. Often, it follows an injury to the joint, and this seems to precipitate a flare-up. The attacks can be extremely painful and lead to severe disability until they are diagnosed and treated.

Sometimes you may think you have arthritis when, in fact, you have *bursitis*. The smooth lining around joints becomes inflamed and causes arthritis-like pain. The condition can be incapacitating, especially when it affects the shoulders. Treatment, sometimes with cortisone injections into the inflamed sac, usually relieves the pain rapidly.

What is polymyalgia rheumatica?

Although often thought of as a type of rheumatism, polymyalgia rheumatica affects the blood vessels rather than the joints. The symptoms, however, are usually aches and pains in the muscles and joints, especially around the shoulders and hips. Sometimes back pain may become severe and result in weakness, which makes it impossible to get out of a chair. The symptoms include weight loss, poor appetite, headache, a sudden loss of vision, and depression. A blood test known as an *erythrocyte sedimentation rate* (ESR) and a *biopsy* of a blood vessel in the scalp may be necessary to diagnose this condition.

This illness should be considered whenever an unusual type of rheumatism occurs. Treatment with cortisone by mouth is usually effective. It may have to be continued for eighteen to twenty-four months, but the dose can be gradually decreased to avoid side effects.

What is the best treatment for arthritis?

The choice of therapy depends on the variety of arthritis and other medical problems that exist at the same time: No single treatment exists for all types.

If you suffer from severe *osteoarthritis* in a large joint, treatment might include heat applied to the affected area and rest and immobilization, either by remaining in bed or using custom-designed splints. Medications that decrease inflammation, such as aspirin or one of the newer antiinflammatory drugs, might be helpful. Very occasionally, injections of cortisone into the joint are valuable, but frequent injections should be avoided. If your hip joint is severely affected and you are incapacitated, surgical replacement might be considered. This can result in a dramatic improvement in your symptoms and in your ability to function.

Rheumatoid arthritis is often treated with large doses of aspirin or other antiinflammatory agents. Special drugs such as gold salts by injection might be used in severe cases. This type of treatment should be supervised by a well-trained specialist in arthritic diseases in conjunction with your family physician. It can be useful if your illness does not respond to other treatments.

347

An episode of acute *gout* can be treated with a course of *colchicine*, taken either by mouth or intravenous injection. Nonaspirin antiinflammatory drugs also usually offer fairly rapid relief of symptoms. Depending on the underlying cause, drugs that decrease the amount of uric acid in the blood can prevent further attacks. Small doses of colchicine taken on a long-term basis may also help decrease your risk of acute attacks of gout.

Pseudogout is treated with antiinflammatory agents as well as injections of cortisone into the joint. Before the joint is injected, fluid is usually removed to make sure that it is not infected. After treatment of a sudden episode of pseudogout, there is usually no need for long-term therapy to prevent further attacks, as opposed to the treatment for gout.

Salicylate, either as plain aspirin or enteric-coated (stomach) aspirin, is probably the single most valuable medication used to treat the various forms of arthritis. Salicylate, in addition to analgesia, decreases inflammation and is most effective when taken regularly four or five times a day, and not only when pain intensifies. As such, it *prevents* pain rather than just *relieving* it.

Some people either cannot tolerate salicylate or do not respond to it. In such cases some antiinflammatory drugs that are different from aspirin and less dangerous than cortisone are now available. There are many different types, and no specific drug appears to be more effective universally than the other. In many instances it is a matter of trial and error to see which preparation works for you.

Gold salts or certain antimalarial drugs have been used in some severe cases of rheumatoid arthritis. Newer medications, like *penicillamine*, are used very occasionally. These work by interfering with the immunological system that somehow appears to keep the disease active. Some people become more prone to infection when they receive medications that affect the immunological system.

Cortisone by mouth is controversial in the treatment of arthritic conditions, especially rheumatoid arthritis. In general, its continued use is avoided because the cumulative side effects, such as weakened bones, bloated appearance, diabetes mellitus, and high blood pressure, can be dangerous. Local injections of cortisone into the painful joint, on the other hand, can be very useful in the treatment of gout, pseudogout, osteoarthritis, and certain cases of rheumatoid arthritis. They can provide immediate relief while you begin another medication, or until you begin a program of physical rehabilitation.

What types of nondrug treatment are useful in the management of arthritic conditions?

Physical therapy, including local heat, massage, whirlpool treatments, shortwave radiation, splinting, mechanical aids, and the retraining of walking habits, may have a place in the management of the various forms of arthritis. In many cases, even though arthritis cannot be cured, the symptoms and the ability to function can be improved by well-directed physical therapy. A competent therapist who is properly trained and experienced in dealing with the elderly should be sought for this type of treatment. Often, the direction of a specialist in arthritic conditions, in addition to a physical therapist, is helpful in designing a suitable program.

When is surgery necessary for an arthritic joint?

Modern medicine has made great advances in the replacement of worn or broken joint components. Once the hip joint has been severely damaged by arthritis, medical treatment may no longer be able to assure comfort and allow reasonable mobility. In such cases you and your physician should consider hip-replacement surgery. The surgery, although major, can be done successfully on most older people, depending on their overall state of health.

A new hip joint is made from a special type of steel, and the parts that touch each other are covered with a synthetic material that allows smooth and easy movement. A unique glue affixes the joint components to the bones. Most people can start to walk within a few days after surgery, although a period of convalescence and rehabilitation may be required before you become fully ambulatory again.

Some people are unduly frightened by the prospect of such surgery, but I have seen many older people who were virtually housebound because of pain return to physically active lives.

BACK PAIN

One of the most common problems affecting people of all ages is back pain. You have only to look around the waiting room of an orthopedist's office to see the number of people suffering from this condition. The fact that back disorders often affect relatively healthy and energetic young people suggests that with increasing age this condition will continue.

The lower back contains the segments of the *vertebral column* (backbone). Within it are nerves that come from the

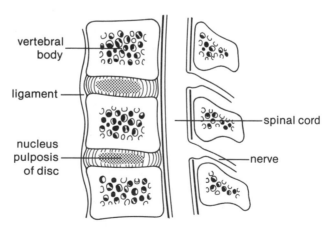

CROSS SECTION OF SPINAL CORD.

spinal cord. The nerves leave the *spinal canal* (the space in the vertebral column) through small outlets between the vertebrae and make their way to the lower part of the abdomen, pelvis, and legs. When the segments of the vertebral column become abnormal, the connecting joints may develop a type of arthritis. Because of this, there may be pressure, causing the nerves to become "pinched."

In youth the vertebral segments are cushioned by discs, a flexible, resilient material called the *nucleus pulposus.* With age the discs become relatively dry and less resilient. Subsequently, the distance between the vertebral segments decreases, and the mobility and flexibility of the spine diminishes.

The *ligaments* supporting the vertebral segments may also become weakened and stretched, leading to a combination of arthritic changes within the vertebral column and a narrowing of the spaces through which the nerves pass. A *slipped disc,* which protrudes and presses on nerves, and other mechanical derangements affecting the spaces between the vertebral bodies and its ligaments can all lead to low back pain.

Other, unusual causes of low back pain must be excluded before your physician assumes that your discomfort is the result of a mechanical imbalance of the vertebral column. Different kinds of tumors can affect bones, including those in the vertebrae, and, although rare, infections affecting the bones *(osteomyelitis)* can also occur. *Paget's disease*, a metabolic process in which the bones recycle calcium at an excessive speed, can affect the backbone and lead to chronic back pain. Other bones, including the pelvis and skull, are frequently afflicted with Paget's disease.

One common cause of abrupt, severe back pain is the sudden *collapse (compression fracture)* of one or more vertebrae. Possibly because of more dramatic changes in hormone balance that occur after the menopause, this is more common in women than in men. There is a progressive "thinning" of bones that often occurs with age. The pain is frequently severe but usually subsides within a few days or weeks.

How is the cause of low back pain diagnosed?

If you have never suffered from back problems and suddenly develop back pain, you should have a physical examination to make sure that the nerves coming from your spinal cord have not been impinged upon by the vertebrae. Your doctor should check your reflexes and the strength and feeling in your legs and feet. He should check to see that your symptoms do not affect your bladder or bowel. Damage to nerves going to these organs can occur if the nerves are pressed upon by tumors or outgrowths from an arthritic spine. Difficulty with urination or diarrhea are warning signs.

The next step should include a plain X-ray of your spine. If the diagnosis is elusive, sometimes a bone scan and special X-rays, such as a *myelogram*, may be needed to determine whether there is excessive pressure on the nerves within the spinal canal.

What is the best treatment for back pain?

If your back pain is the result of a tumor in the bones, you will no doubt require surgery, special drugs, or radiation therapy, alone or in combination. Illnesses such as Paget's disease are presently treated with medications that decrease the metabolic activity within the bones and relieve the pain. A sudden compression fracture usually causes severe pain, which subsides on its own within a few days of bed rest, applied heat, and pain medications.

After the physician has exhausted other possibilities, he will probably conclude that the back pain is the result of a derangement of your vertebral column and its joints and ligaments. This may become increasingly severe as you grow older.

Treatment will be successful only if you cooperate with your physician and follow the principles that will improve the mechanics of your vertebral column and retrain the muscles controlling it. Many medical clinics are specifically organized for the care of back pain. Your physician may refer you to one of these clinics, or he may recommend treatment himself.

The first step of treatment is to lose weight so that there is less strain on your backbone. If your pain is severe, you may require a period of complete bed rest in order to relax the muscle spasms. Muscle relaxants and analgesics are often used during this period. Heat directly applied to your back may be helpful. Quite frequently, traction done in a hospital or a physical therapy clinic is employed. This pulls on the upper and lower parts of your spine and may relieve muscle spasm.

The real solution to solving low back pain is to learn how to change your posture and the way you lie, lift, bend, sit, and walk. You should learn the various exercises that strengthen the muscles supporting your back. It is important that you bend at the knees, rather than with your back, when you lift something. You may have to change the way you carry packages. This is especially important when you shop in a supermarket. I recommend that you ask the checkout clerk to pack your items in more bags than usual so that each bag weighs less and is more easily lifted. Try to lift them with your arms, rather than with your back, in order to avoid strain. Sudden twisting motions should be avoided. It is usually worthwhile to get a firm mattress. When you experience pain or discomfort you should raise your legs slightly on a few pillows or bend your knees when you are lying flat on your back in bed. It is often more comfortable to lie on your side with your legs slightly bent and your back curled.

Exercises to improve your muscle tone should also be learned. Once your symptoms improve, you could take up swimming, which strengthens your muscles and relieves the tension on your vertebral column. Sometimes a specially designed corset may be of value, not only in relieving pain, but to prevent you from bending your back in ways that will aggravate your pain and discomfort.

Sometimes the pressure on the nerves is so great that you

may experience pain similar to *intermittent claudication* (see page 212) when you walk, and weakness and progressive disability in your legs may occur. Such circumstances usually require a *myelogram* in order to determine whether your spinal canal has narrowed. If your symptoms become more pronounced or if you develop problems with your bladder and bowel, surgery may be necessary to relieve the pressure. In most instances the surgery is effective and successful and will result in an improvement in your symptoms. Surgery on the back should be avoided if it is being done for back pain only. It is often not successful in this situation and usually is reserved for those cases where there is damaging pressure on nerves.

Some older women with very thin bones *(osteoporosis)* suffer from frequent compression fractures. They often have severe back pain and may get little relief from rest and exercise alone. Some physicians prescribe vitamin D and calcium supplements in these circumstances. Not everyone gains relief, but it is worth a try. Your physician will check for signs of excess calcium accumulation as an unwanted side effect after this treatment has begun.

In many instances a carefully followed program of weight reduction, changes in posture and movements, and a well-designed exercise program can relieve your pain and allow you to return to normal physical activities in comfort. Rarely is surgery necessary. It should be considered only after a more conservative approach has been tried, unless there is severe pressure on nerves. Then it may be necessary in order to avoid permanent damage to nerves, which can lead to irreversible weakness or urinary incontinence.

Can a chiropractor be helpful?

Physicians usually have a rather negative attitude about the manipulations performed by chiropractors. However, many patients think very highly of the care they have received from them. It is often difficult to discount relief from pain, which seems to occur miraculously at the hands of chiropractors.

All the methods used by chiropractors to achieve their results are difficult to evaluate completely. Some physicians specializing in rehabilitation or orthopedics and a number of physiotherapists have learned the techniques of manipulation practiced by chiropractors and employ them judiciously in some patients.

My main concern about the consultation of chiropractors by the elderly is that many problems can cause back pain or other types of joint pain. If, by chance, a manipulation is performed on the back of a person with a serious disease other than a mechanical derangement, severe damage can occur. The thinner bones of the elderly are also more prone to injury that may occur from inappropriate manipulations. Damage to nerves is more likely in the elderly if manipulations are carried out when nerves are being pressed upon by parts of the vertebrae.

You may continue to go to a chiropractor despite the advice of your physician. This is especially so if you have experienced prompt relief from back discomfort after your chiropractic treatment. If your pain is not relieved as quickly as usual, however, I would recommend getting a medical opinion in order to verify that the pain is not from another disorder, the treatment of which might *not* be chiropractic manipulation.

BROKEN BONES

Some older individuals seem to have a tendency to break bones. Falling and the broken bones resulting from falls are more common as you grow older. Although other bones may break, such as the bones of the spine and the arm, the most common broken bone in the elderly is the hip. Sometimes a bone may break without much trauma or stress, or you may fall and break your hip and assume that the fall caused the break. In many cases the break occurs spontaneously because of bone brittleness and leads to the fall, often without much pain.

How is a broken hip treated?

If you break your hip, the chances are you will suffer from pain and not be able to walk. Sometimes a hip will break in such a way that the two broken ends become impacted, and you may be able to walk on the leg without much pain. This is rare, however. Most people are unable to walk unless the hip is repaired surgically.

The dangers of surgery are outweighed by the dangers that are inherent in remaining bedridden for a prolonged period. There is an increased risk of serious illnesses such as pneumonia, phlebitis, and urinary tract infections, and the health of the skin may be difficult to maintain when bedridden. Also, the psychological effect of being bedridden is extremely negative.

Most surgeons use a metal device to hold the broken hip in place. Sometimes a pin is put in to connect the ball of the hip joint with the shaft of the thigh bone. Occasionally, the surgeon may have to replace the ball of the joint with a metal one. If you have had hip surgery, in most instances you should be out of bed within a few days and able to begin a physical rehabilitation program.

During the past year I have treated a number of very elderly ladies, all over 90, who suffered from hip fractures. Every one had hip surgery and returned to full independence in less than three months.

CHAPTER 18

Endocrine (Hormone Gland) Abnormalities

The endocrine glands, distributed throughout the body produce *hormones*, which help to control the chemical reactions of the body's cells. We often use the word *metabolism* to describe the different cell processes. The most important endocrine glands are the *thyroid gland*, the two *adrenal glands*, the *pancreas*, the four *parathyroid glands*, and the *pituitary gland*. The *sex glands* (ovaries and testicles) also produce hormones, but they are usually considered separately from the endocrine system.

Each of the endocrine glands produces its own special hormone or hormones, which help keep the cells of the body functioning properly and efficiently. When an endocrine gland becomes diseased, it may produce too much or too little of its hormone and upset the body's metabolism. In most cases the diseases that develop are treatable.

THE THYROID GLAND

The thyroid gland, found in the neck just below the Adam's apple, is shaped like a butterfly, with each of the wings called the thyroid *lobes*. The thyroid gland produces *thyroid hormone (thyroxine)*, a substance necessary for metabolism.

Certain blood tests measure the amount of thyroid hormone in the blood and help in diagnosis. It is sometimes necessary to do a *radioactive thyroid uptake and scan* in order to diagnose some thyroid disorders completely. In many instances thyroid disease requires repeated tests. Unfortunately, disease of the thyroid gland can be very subtle as you grow older. Both overactivity and underactivity can be confused with other conditions. For this reason diagnosis and successful treatment are frequently and unnecessarily delayed.

HYPERTHYROIDISM (OVERACTIVE THYROID GLAND)

Hyperthyroidism affects many parts of the body, especially the heart. If you already suffer from a heart condition, the increased hormone, which causes the heart to speed up, can aggravate heart failure and cause irregular heart rhythms.

Mood changes, such as agitation, mental confusion, apathy, and depression, can occur, as well as weight loss (despite a good appetite) and a change in bowel habits, with a tendency toward diarrhea. You may begin to prefer cold weather and find that you are constantly opening windows when the rest of your family is closing them. There may be a shaking of your hands, which may make you think that you are excessively "nervous." Indeed, you may become more nervous and irritable for no reason. Because many of these symptoms are vague, the condition may not be immediately suspected. The diagnosis is confirmed by blood tests that measure the excess amount of thyroid hormone in the blood.

What is the treatment for hyperthyroidism?

Once a diagnosis is made, treatment is usually successful. Excess thyroid hormone can be corrected with medications, and improvement can be seen quickly so long as the drugs are taken. Medications such as *propylthiouracil* block the manufacture of thyroid hormone. *Beta-blockers*, also used to treat angina pectoris and high blood pressure, effectively blunt the effects of excess thyroid hormone on the heart. These drugs, however, do not correct the underlying cause of the excess thyroid hormone production, but they do correct the symptoms while other treatment is being planned.

The underlying cause of hyperthyroidism is treated frequently with *radioactive iodine*, taken by mouth. Thyroid-blocking medications may be necessary for a while after the radioactive iodine is given. Eventually, the radioactive treatment has a permanent effect, and the other medications are discontinued.

Is there any danger to treatment?

The medications and the radioactive therapy have few serious side effects. In very rare cases some thyroid-blocking drugs can cause problems with the bone marrow.

The most common problem that can occur after treatment with radioactive iodine is that the thyroid gland may become underactive. This is frequently unavoidable, but correction is easy, and your physician will check for this periodically.

HYPOTHYROIDISM (UNDERACTIVE THYROID GLAND)

Hypothyroidism usually develops very gradually. The main symptom is a general slowing down, both mentally and physically. You may experience some memory impairment, fatigue, weight gain, and a slowing of your bowel habits. Some people notice a deepening of their voice. You may find that you always feel cold and notice some dryness of your skin. Sometimes you will develop symptoms of heart disease, especially if you suffer from angina pectoris or heart failure.

These symptoms are commonly considered to be the unavoidable consequence of aging, so unless hypothyroidism is considered, your treatment may be unnecessarily delayed. The older, untreated hypothyroid person gradually gets slower and slower, and duller and duller. As a result, the person is usually too sluggish and mentally impaired to look after himself.

If you are hypothyroid and at the same time suffer from another illness, the diagnosis could be missed because the emphasis may be directed to the other condition. An elderly gentleman whom I saw was admitted to the hospital because of a stroke. During the next three months all the effort was put into rehabilitating him so that he would be well enough to go home. Just before his discharge, he developed swelling of his legs. He was found to have a hoarse voice, and dry skin, and he was not as alert as other stroke victims.

When his underactive thyroid gland was treated, his mind improved remarkably. The swelling of his legs disappeared, and he was able to manage almost completely independently, other than needing the assistance of a walker. During his hospitalization the stroke took such precedence that the symptoms of hypothyroidism were overlooked until they became advanced. In fact, the recovery from his stroke was impaired until his hypothyroidism was treated.

Is treatment dangerous?

The main problem in the treatment of hypothyroidism is that you may also have heart disease. If your thyroid disease is treated too quickly, your heart disease may worsen. In this case thyroid hormone replacement is recommended, starting with very small doses and increasing them gradually.

It may take as long as four to six months of treatment for you to reach normal thyroid function, although the good effects begin to be felt within two or three months. By increasing the dosage slowly, the dangerous effects can be avoided. It is unusual for you to receive too much thyroid hormone, because periodic blood tests determine the right amount of medication.

Can treatment ever be stopped?

Once a diagnosis of hypothyroidism is made, thyroid hormone replacement has to be continued for the rest of your life. But if it is stopped for a few days, it can be started again at the same dosage. If, by chance, it is stopped for a few weeks or longer, it should be restarted more gradually and increased back to full dosage slowly. Your physician will determine the correct dosage and speed. You should not restart your medication at full strength without his advice if many weeks have elapsed.

THE ADRENAL GLANDS

The *adrenal glands* produce the hormone *cortisone*, which controls the amount of fluid and salt in the body and helps the body respond to *stress*. The correct amount of cortisone is important for your feeling of well-being. Some illnesses affecting older people can lead to a decrease in the spontaneous production of cortisone. However, most cases of insufficient natural cortisone occur because a cortisone medication has been prescribed which suppresses the body's need to produce its own.

Some people spontaneously produce excess amounts of cortisone, which leads to *Cushing's disease*. The cortisone accumulates and adversely affects many parts of the body.

Why do some people stop producing normal amounts of cortisone?

There are some illnesses in which the adrenal glands stop working partially or completely. They can be affected by a tuberculosis infection or by a tumor. Or the glands shut off for no apparent reason.

If you lack cortisone, you will probably feel weak and have

361

little energy. You may lose weight or be found to have low blood pressure. The color of your skin may darken even when you have not been in the sun. Nausea, loss of appetite, and frequent vomiting also can occur. The natural illness, known as *Addison's disease*, progresses slowly, but it may become serious under stressful situations. If, for instance, you require surgery and an anesthetic, a lack of cortisone can lead to severe complications. Any physician or surgeon should be aware that you suffer from Addison's disease so that cortisone can be given before surgery.

The diagnosis is made through blood tests, which will show if the *electrolytes* are abnormal and if the amount of cortisone is sufficient. Treatment is with cortisone, usually given as pills. The medication must be continued for life.

If you are receiving cortisone by injection or pills for illnesses such as asthma or rheumatoid arthritis, the adrenal glands may become underactive. In effect, they "think" that they have sufficient cortisone and therefore shut off their own production. If you stop taking the cortisone medication suddenly, they do not have enough time to produce their own supply to replace the lost cortisone. This leads to a drop in blood pressure, general weakness, and often nausea and vomiting. If left untreated, it can lead to shock just as in Addison's disease.

What precautions should you take if you are receiving cortisone by pills or injections, or know that you have Addison's disease?

It is important for you to wear a wrist bracelet that says you are receiving cortisone therapy. These bracelets are available through organizations such as *Medic-Alert*, which also keep a record of your illness and treatment.

The main danger is that during a serious illness, infection, or surgery, your body may not be able to produce enough cortisone to meet the body's requirements. Because your adrenal glands have shut off, you may go into shock because of the stress. A new physician in an emergency situation will check your bracelet and temporarily increase the amount of cortisone.

What happens when the adrenal glands produce too much cortisone?

Very rarely, a person develops a tumor of the adrenal glands, which causes an overproduction of cortisone. You may become overweight and develop high blood pressure or diabetes mellitus. Your bones may weaken and be prone to fractures, and your skin may develop small hemorrhages under the surface at the slightest touch. You may begin to feel generally weak and ill.

The diagnosis is made by special blood tests. Treatment may consist of surgical removal of one or both adrenal glands. In many cases radiation to the *pituitary gland* can be effective in halting the disease. The pituitary gland is located in the brain and manufactures the hormone ACTH, which stimulates the adrenal gland to produce cortisone. Radiation can sometimes stop the formation of excess amounts of ACTH, thus decreasing the amount of cortisone.

Too much cortisone medication can cause the same symptoms. When cortisone treatment is required, as in rheumatoid arthritis or asthma, the pills sometimes can be taken every two days instead of every day to decrease some of the side effects. Your physician can monitor your treatment and check the effects.

DIABETES MELLITUS

In *diabetes mellitus* the body's blood sugar control becomes impaired. This should be differentiated from *diabetes insipidus*, an illness of the pituitary gland, in which excess urine is passed. A great deal of urine is also passed in diabetes mellitus, but the urine contains a large amount of sugar (glucose).

The amount of glucose in your blood is determined by a

number of factors. The different types of carbohydrates that are ingested are converted into *glucose*, a simple sugar that stimulates the pancreas to increase its output of the hormone *insulin*. Insulin helps the body metabolize carbohydrates, converting nutrients into glucose. The manner in which glucose and other nutrients are used by your body is also governed by the amount of insulin produced. The amount of glucose in your blood varies with the amount of food that you eat and the amount of exercise that you do.

If there is too little insulin, the level of glucose in your blood rises. If the glucose reaches a certain level, it begins to leak through the kidneys and "spills" into your urine. Many physicians teach their patients how to measure the amount of glucose in the urine with special tablets or "tapes" to see if it is too high.

As you grow older, your pancreas may become less able to produce enough insulin to fill your needs. If you are overweight, you may be putting an extra load on your pancreas. Even though there appears to be enough insulin, its effect is impaired because of the excess weight.

The most common type of diabetes mellitus in older individuals is called *adult onset* diabetes. This may affect you much more gradually than the kind that begins in younger people. Although it is not quite so dangerous, it must be treated carefully and controlled properly in order to avoid complications.

Why might you "develop" diabetes when you receive certain medications or suffer from other illnesses?

Many people have what is called *latent diabetes mellitus*. This means that your body has trouble controlling the blood glucose level. This may not become obvious until you take certain medications or experience certain stressful illnesses. You do not develop the diabetes mellitus *because* of the medications or illness, but you have a tendency toward it, and it manifests itself for the first time under these stressful circumstances. It may manifest itself during a heart attack or pneumonia, for example. *Diuretics* and *cortisone* may cause diabetes to become evident.

How is diabetes mellitus diagnosed?

The symptoms of diabetes mellitus are the need to pass urine frequently or recurrent urinary tract infections. A vaginal yeast infection, with severe itching is often a sign of diabetes in older women. You may become excessively thirsty and feel generally ill, with some weight loss and a decreased appetite. However, if you are overweight, you may not have the last symptoms. In fact, your weight and appetite may increase. Some people notice trouble with their vision or feel dizzy.

Your blood glucose may be high and consequently spill into your urine, which increases your chance of a urinary tract infection. The high blood and urine glucose levels are usually enough to make a diagnosis. Sometimes, to confirm the diagnosis, a *glucose tolerance test* may be needed, which shows whether your body is controlling its blood glucose normally. Latent diabetes mellitus may also be uncovered by this test.

What is the best treatment?

Relatively few older people are required to begin insulin treatment to control their diabetes. If you have suffered from diabetes for many years, you may already be taking insulin, however.

Many older people can have their blood glucose levels lowered by medications that stimulate the pancreas to produce more insulin. These medications are controversial, however, because recent studies suggest that they increase the risk of ischemic heart disease (angina pectoris, myocardial infarction).

The main thrust of diabetic control is to lose weight. In the vast majority of older individuals, adequate weight loss will eliminate the need for pills to control blood glucose levels. In those who find weight loss difficult, it may be necessary to take the medications despite the small risk of heart disease. If more people realized the increased risk of heart disease from these medications, they would be more careful with their diets.

How important is a diabetic diet?

In many cases diet alone is sufficient to control the symptoms of diabetes mellitus and bring your blood glucose back to normal. For those people receiving *insulin*, diet is even more important in order to control the balance between insulin and glucose levels. Some physicians recommend a very strict diet, whereas others are more tolerant. It is sometimes difficult for the older person to achieve strict control of his diabetes when insulin is required. Moderate control is probably the best approach in older persons. It is safer than very strict control which demands that sugar levels stay on the low side, because an excessively low blood glucose can be dangerous.

For those who do not require insulin, the goal should be to reduce food intake and reduce and maintain your "ideal weight." Cutting out sugar is not sufficient for a diabetic diet. Your body is able to turn all foods into glucose and fat if they are eaten in large enough quantities. A balanced, limited-calorie diet is essential. Your physician or a dietitian can help you learn the principles of a diabetic diet. With good dietary management your symptoms can be controlled, your glucose levels brought back to normal, and in many instances the use of pills avoided. It takes willpower and knowledge, but it is worth the effort.

What are the dangers of diabetes?

Diabetics are in greater danger of developing infections, especially of the urinary tract. They also develop narrowing of the blood vessels as a result of *atherosclerosis*. This can result in an increased tendency to strokes, ischemic heart disease, peripheral vascular disease, kidney ailments, and eye disease. It

366

appears that if care is taken to control the diabetes, the risk of these complications decreases.

Diabetics may develop ischemic heart disease without the usual symptoms of chest pain, and a heart attack (myocardial infarction) also may be experienced without chest pain and be revealed incidentally on a cardiogram long after the attack occurred.

If you are diabetic, you should take great care of your feet. Your nails should be cut properly (straight across) with the assistance of a physician, podiatrist, or chiropodist. Any foot infection or injury must be treated immediately to prevent progression and the possible risk of impaired blood supply and gangrene.

Can diabetes be cured?

In most instances the illness cannot be cured, but it can be well controlled. If you have latent diabetes mellitus, which becomes evident when taking medications such as diuretics or cortisone, stopping the drugs may result in your blood glucose returning to normal. This is not a cure, but a return to the latent state. If this is the case, the diabetes may recur in the future. It is therefore important to watch your diet and your weight and have periodic medical supervision.

How should diabetes treatment be followed?

You should control your diet and weight, using the guidelines suggested by your physician. If you are receiving insulin or pills, it is important to learn how to examine your urine periodically to see if glucose is spilling into it. Your physician will usually arrange for periodic (two-three months) blood glucose tests to see if it is under control. A more extensive physical examination every six months should be done to maintain careful glucose control and to check your eyes, feet, urine, blood pressure, and heart in particular. Seeing an eye specialist once a year is helpful in recognizing and treating diabetic eye disease.

OTHER ENDOCRINE DISORDERS

The *pituitary gland*, in the brain, produces different hormones that control the function of other endocrine glands in the body. It regulates and monitors their normal hormone production. For example, the adrenal glands produce cortisone according to the amount of the stimulating hormone ACTH from the pituitary gland. This is also the case with the thyroid and sex glands.

Sometimes the pituitary gland enlarges and a tumor develops. The result may be an excess of one hormone or pressure on the brain or on the optic nerves. The results may be a loss of vision if the tumor is not discovered and treated in time. Occasionally, the gland may not produce enough of a certain hormone, and a hormone deficiency disease results. If, for instance, the thyroid stimulating hormone is not produced, you may develop hypothyroidism. Although the illness looks similar to the other, more common, type of hypothyroidism due to disease of the thyroid gland itself, it should be recognized because other pituitary hormones may also fail. The function of the pituitary gland is determined by special blood tests that measure the production of the stimulating hormones.

The four small glands just behind the thyroid gland, known as the *parathyroid glands*, regulate the amount of calcium and phosphorus in the blood. The balance of these substances depends on the amount received in the diet, lost by the kidneys, and stored in the bones. The *parathyroid hormone (parathormone)* governs the interaction of the food absorption, bone formation, and loss through the urine. As a result, the amount of calcium and phosphorus in the blood is kept closely in check. If the parathyroid glands become overactive you may develop excess amounts of calcium in your blood and urine.

The symptoms include mental confusion, the need to pass large amounts of urine, the formation of kidney stones, and pain in the bones. Ulcer disease of the stomach occurs more often.

The diagnosis is often difficult to make because endocrine disorders of this type are rare in older people. A raised calcium level may be found by chance during routine blood tests. If no other symptoms are present, blood tests every few months will show if the calcium level is becoming unduly high. If, however, you have symptoms of parathyroid hormone excess, the parathyroid glands must be removed surgically. In general, the outlook for this surgery is very good.

HYPOGLYCEMIA (LOW BLOOD SUGAR)

Rarely, the insulin-producing glands within the pancreas develop a tumor and produce too much insulin, which causes the blood glucose to become low. This is called *hypoglycemia*, often referred to as *low blood sugar*. You may have frequent episodes of mental confusion, giddiness, dizziness, or fainting. The diagnosis is made by finding extremely low blood glucose levels. Surgical removal of the insulin-producing tumor usually results in a cure. The tumor itself is most often benign and will not spread or return once it is removed.

A great deal has been written recently about *spontaneous hypoglycemia* as a possible cause of many emotional problems, especially in younger people. Whether this is true in the older individual is not certain, but it seems to be much less common, if it exists at all. Insulin-producing tumors are very rarely found in people considered to be suffering from spontaneous hypoglycemia. In some overweight people who have latent diabetes mellitus, there may be a transient period of hypoglycemia a few hours after a large carbohydrate-rich meal. The best treatment for this condition is to lose weight and decrease the intake of carbohydrates.

Diabetes insipidus is an uncommon ailment in the elderly. It is the result of a lack of *antidiuretic hormone*, or ADH, produced by the pituitary gland. The main symptoms are constant thirst and the passage of large amounts of urine. In the early stages it may be mistaken for diabetes mellitus, but a blood test and urine test of the glucose level will easily differentiate these two illnesses. It can be treated with injections of the hormone, which are given every few days.

CHAPTER 19

Hematological (Blood) Disorders

Blood consists of *plasma*, a fluid that carries red blood cells *(erythrocytes)* and white blood cells *(leucocytes)*. Red blood cells carry oxygen and carbon dixoide, which are necessary for respiration and metabolism, whereas white cells protect the body from infection. Many elements are contained in the plasma, including important salts, proteins, antibodies, nutrients, and many byproducts of metabolism. *Platelets* are small cell-like particles that help the blood clot when there is an injury to a blood vessel.

The diseases of the blood that can affect older people are the result of a decrease in the red or white blood cells or an increase of blood cells that may not be working normally. Another problem includes a decrease in the *clotting* ability of the blood, which can lead to abnormal bruising or bleeding. Sometimes the opposite occurs: The blood may clot *(thrombose)* within normal blood vessels for no apparent reason and deprive a part of the body of its blood supply.

ANEMIA

One common problem that may affect you in your later years is *anemia*, which means that the amount of red blood cells in the body is reduced and therefore the ability to carry oxygen and carbon dioxide is impaired. Oxygen is essential for normal activities: When the blood carries less of it, the body loses its energy and becomes easily tired.

For your red blood cells to develop and function normally, you need *iron* and certain vitamins, including *vitamin B_{12}* and *folic acid*. A lack of adequate amounts of these elements can cause anemia.

It is often assumed by older people that being anemic is a natural consequence of aging, that some degree of fatigue and lack of pep is normal. This attitude may be shared by members of your family and even by some members of the medical profession. But unless you have a specific illness causing anemia, your blood count should not be much less than that of a younger person. If it is lower, the cause should be looked for and treated. It should *never* be accepted as a consequence of aging alone.

Do you need extra iron to prevent anemia?

Normally the body loses relatively little iron, except in women who are still menstruating. The amount of iron that is naturally lost through the bowel and skin is quite small. Thus you should need no more iron than a younger person. If you are found to have too little iron in your blood cells, it usually means that there is an unrecognized source of bleeding, often in the bowel.

Occasionally an older person may have an iron-poor diet, containing virtually no meat or protein. This could account for a mild degree of iron-deficiency (low iron) anemia. This is less likely in Western countries, but it does occur occasionally in elderly people who are poor or who have been vegetarians for many years.

Iron should not be taken as a "tonic." If an iron-deficiency anemia is discovered, you should undergo a full investigation, especially of your diet and your intestinal tract. Treatment does not have to be withheld while the anemia is being investigated. However, even though you may feel better after you receive iron therapy or blood transfusions, a proper evaluation should not be postponed.

Sometimes the cause of an iron-deficiency anemia can be mysterious and elusive, frustrating both the physician and the patient. One 91-year-old lady was referred to me because she complained about having suffered from anemia for more than ten years. The anemia would come and go, sometimes getting better with iron pills and sometimes not. She had had many X-rays of her gastrointestinal tract as well as a *gastroscopy* and *colonoscopy*, but no cause was found. However, when her stools were checked, they revealed microscopic amounts of blood. Sometimes she noticed small amounts of red blood in the toilet bowl, but this happened infrequently.

Now, at 91, her anemia had become so bad that she required periodic blood transfusions because iron therapy alone no longer kept her blood count high enough to avoid constant fatigue. Because the other X-rays were unrevealing, I resorted to an *angiogram* of her intestines to determine whether a source of bleeding had been overlooked. When I asked the radiologist to do this X-ray, which does have some risk, he looked at me as though I were crazy and said, "She's 91. Why don't we just leave her alone and treat her with blood transfusions?" I persisted in my request for the X-ray and told him that she had to attend the wedding of a great-granddaughter in a few weeks. He reluctantly agreed to do the angiogram, which indeed did reveal that she was bleeding from a small blood vessel in her large bowel. Within a few days she had bowel surgery and was found to have a benign abnormality of blood vessels that made them leak frequently, thereby causing her to be anemic. She withstood the surgery remarkably well, left the hospital in ten days, and was able to attend the wedding. Now, at 93, she continues to be well, without anemia, more than two years after her surgery.

What is pernicious anemia?

Pernicious anemia is caused by the lack of a substance in the stomach *(intrinsic factor)* that is needed to absorb vitamin B_{12}. The resultant lack of vitamin B_{12} causes anemia, as well as problems with the nervous system. *Vitamin B_{12}* helps in the formation of normal red blood cells. Before the discovery of the cause and treatment of this anemia, it was indeed pernicious. Many older people became progressively ill, anemic, and weak, and eventually died.

Pernicious anemia can occur in older people with thyroid disease or in those who have undergone some type of stomach or intestinal surgery. Sometimes it occurs spontaneously, and it occasionally runs in families. You may feel weak and short of breath and have nervous system symptoms, such as tingling in the feet, difficulty in balance, and some memory loss. The diagnosis is made with blood tests and special types of urine tests that measure the absorption of vitamin B_{12}. A *bone marrow biopsy* also is often helpful.

Treatment is relatively simple: It consists of injections of vitamin B_{12}, which are given once a month. Many individuals who may have assumed that their weakness and fatigue were part of aging are happily surprised after they receive vitamin B_{12} injections. If you do not have a vitamin B_{12} deficiency, though, injections will not make you feel stronger, so you should not take the vitamin for an energy "boost," as was done many years ago.

One elderly lady who lived in a nursing home had always been very active and well-read. She was asked if she would like to work in the residents' library. Unexpectedly, she declined, saying that she recently had had difficulty concentrating while reading. Her attending physician became suspicious and invited her for a medical examination. Careful questioning revealed that she became a little short of breath when she walked and had to hold onto the wall because she was afraid of falling.

Tests revealed that she had a low vitamin B_{12} level and was quite anemic. A year before, her blood count was only somewhat lower than normal, but at the time further investigations had not been done. After she was treated with vitamin B_{12}, her blood count bounced back to normal and all of her symptoms disappeared. She now runs the library full-time and can not only tell you where the books are, but she seems to have read almost all of them.

What other vitamin is needed for "healthy" blood?

Folic acid is another vitamin that is required for your body to produce normal blood. This vitamin is found in green vegetables but is easily destroyed when they are boiled. Some people who do not eat fresh vegetables, especially salad greens, are at a greater risk of developing a deficiency of this vitamin. Excess alcohol use and the administration of certain drugs, such as *phenytoin* (Dilantin®) used in epilepsy, can also cause folic acid deficiency. The anemia caused by a lack of folic acid is similar to pernicious anemia, but it usually improves with folic acid supplements.

What other kinds of anemia can occur?

There are various causes of anemia that are more common in older people. Sometimes the body "breaks down" (hemolyzes) its own red blood cells as if they didn't belong, and the bone marrow (the factory where blood cells are made) cannot keep up with the destruction. The result is *hemolytic anemia*. If you have a chronic disease such as arthritis, kidney disease, or a malignant tumor, your body may not be able to make a normal amount of blood. Certain types of malignancies that affect the blood cells, such as *leukemia*, can also cause anemia.

Each type of anemia requires special tests to find its cause and decide on appropriate treatment. A *bone marrow biopsy* may be necessary to diagnose it. The procedure has no danger and usually causes no pain.

LEUKEMIA AND MULTIPLE MYELOMA

Many blood malignancies progress very slowly in older people. The common malignancies are *chronic leukemia* and *multiple myeloma*, both of which may first reveal themselves as anemia (see page 315). Multiple myeloma sometimes causes bone pain and spontaneous bone fractures. Treatment can usually be accomplished successfully with drugs and occasionally with *radiation therapy*. Proper treatment can bring you to a satisfactory level of well-being and activity and keep you going for a long time.

An 88-year-old gentleman was known to suffer from chronic leukemia for about 25 years. He was active and productive all this time and visited his physician periodically for examinations. In his later years he occasionally required a small degree of *chemotherapy* to keep his leukemia under control. However, at 88, he developed pain in his spleen, which had become enlarged because of the leukemia. Radiation therapy to his spleen improved his symptoms. Some months later, his leukemia began to progress rapidly, and his family came from out of town to prepare themselves for his last days.

His condition was evaluated by a *hematologist* (blood specialist), who recommended a new course of chemotherapy. Beyond anyone's expectations, his white blood-cell count returned to normal, his anemia improved, and he felt well again. Although only a few months have passed since his treatment began, he continues to feel well and enjoy life. His family returned to their homes, and even though everyone is aware of the likelihood of a relapse, he has managed thus far to improve with treatment.

POLYCYTHEMIA

In this condition the body appears to make too much blood rather than too little. In some ways it is the opposite of anemia. However, rather than feeling much better than a person with a normal blood count, you will probably feel weak and tired. You may experience headaches and develop high blood pressure because the blood becomes stickier than normal. There is an increased tendency for blood clots to form, and this can lead to *thrombosis* in any organ of the body.

Treatment usually consists of removing some of the excess blood *(phlebotomy)* every few weeks or giving a radioactive drug that stops the bone marrow from producing the extra blood. There is a risk of strokes and damage to the heart and kidneys. Some people improve with medications such as aspirin, which decreases the stickiness of the blood. You should be followed carefully by your physician or hematologist, who is experienced in dealing with this disease. Most older people with this disorder can be kept healthy for many years with treatment.

INDEX

378